·lth Li

MODELS
FOR
NURSING

MODELS FOR NURSING

Edited by
BETTY KERSHAW MSc SRN RCNT RNT DANS OND
Director of Nursing Studies
Royal Marsden Hospital
London and Sutton

and

JANE SALVAGE BA RGN
Editor, *Senior Nurse*

With 15 contributors

An H M & M Nursing Publication

JOHN WILEY & SONS
Chichester · New York · Brisbane · Toronto · Singapore

H M + M is an imprint of John Wiley & Sons Ltd

Library of Congress Cataloging in Publication Data:

Main entry under title:
Models for nursing.
  (An H M + M nursing publication)
  Includes index.
  1. Nursing—Philosophy. I. Kershaw, Betty.
II. Salvage, Jane. III. Series: H M + M nursing publication.
[DNLM: 1. Models, Theoretical. 2. Nursing Process. WY 100 M6885]
RT84.5.M63 1986   610.73   85–29600
ISBN 0 471 90991 2 (pbk.)

British Library Cataloguing in Publication Data:

Models for nursing.—(An H M + M nursing publication)
  1. Nursing
  I. Kershaw, Betty II. Salvage, Jane
  610.73   RT41

  ISBN 0 471 90991 2

Typeset by Woodfield Graphics, Fontwell, Arundel, West Sussex

Printed and bound in Great Britain by
Biddles Ltd, Guildford and King's Lynn

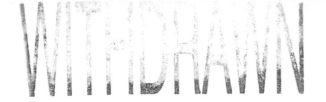

Contributors

GEORGE CASTLEDINE MSc BA DipSocStud SRN FRCN is Principal Lecturer and Consultant in Nursing, a joint appointment between the health authorities of North Wales and the North East Wales Institute of Higher Education.

HUGH CHADDERTON BEd SRN RMN DipN RCNT RNT is Lecturer in the Department of Nursing Studies, University of Glasgow.

JUNE CLARK PhD MPhil BA SRN HVCert DipSocRes FRCN is a senior nurse with Lewisham and North Southwark Health Authority.

BLAIR COLLISTER MSc DANS DipN RMN SRN RCNT RNT is a lecturer in nursing in the Department of Nursing, University of Manchester.

ELIZABETH FARMER RGN SCM DN is Clinical Nurse Manager at Kirklandside Hospital, Hurlford, Kilmarnock.

BETTY KERSHAW MSc SRN RCNT RNT DANS OND is Director of Nursing Studies at the Royal Marsden Hospital, London and Surrey.

WINIFRED LOGAN MA DNS(Educ) RGN RNT is Head of the Department of Health and Nursing Studies, Glasgow College of Technology.

JEAN McFARLANE DSc MSc BSc SRN SCM HVTutCert FRCN, Baroness McFarlane of Llandaff, is Professor and Head of the Department of Nursing, University of Manchester.

ALAN PEARSON PhD MSc RGN ONC RNT Dip NEd DANS FRCN is Senior Nurse, Clinical Practice Development, in the Burford and Oxford Nursing Development Units, Oxfordshire.

NANCY ROPER MPhil RSCN RGN RNT is a self-employed nursing author and lecturer.

JANE SALVAGE BA RGN is a freelance journalist and lecturer; she is editor of the monthly journal *Senior Nurse*.

ALISON TIERNEY BSc PhD RGN is Director of the Nursing Research Unit in the Department of Nursing Studies, University of Edinburgh.

BARBARA VAUGHAN SRN DipN MSc is Senior Tutor, Clinical Practice Development, at the John Radcliffe Hospital, Oxford.

MIKE WALSH BA SRN CertEd is Lecturer in Nursing at Bristol Polytechnic.

STEVE WRIGHT MSc SRN RCNT RNT DipN DANS is Clinical Nurse Specialist in the Care of the Elderly Unit, Tameside General Hospital, Lancashire.

Contents

Preface

Interest in nursing theories and models and the applications of these models to clinical practice has, in the last two years, accelerated in the UK. This book is a result of that growth and has, in part, been prepared to ensure that those nurses who have been unable to attend the relevant conferences nevertheless have access to the work on models being conducted by experienced British nurses.

The chapters reflect not only the growing interest in nursing theory as a foundation for practice, but also the ability of British nurses to study and digest work carried out abroad – primarily in the USA – and to build on it and adapt from it to suit the often very different working conditions at home. We may have started later than our transatlantic colleagues, for they have been evolving their theories for 30 years, but this book suggests that we shall not be slow in catching up. Moreover, it is a sign of great strength that all the contributions in this book have firm roots in and make constant reference back to practice. This is not a claim which could be upheld by all the American theorists.

The pressing need for British nurses to learn, share and develop their thinking on models for and of nursing led us to organise a major conference, run jointly by *Senior Nurse* and the Royal College of Nursing and held in the spring of 1985 at the department of nursing studies in the University of Manchester, with the kind assistance of Professor Baroness McFarlane of Llandaff. The subsequent demand for papers, and the disappointment of those who had to be turned away, prompted us to make them available more widely. This book is the fruit: most of the contributions are based on the conference papers, revised and adapted for publication, with one or two extra ones commissioned to ensure the balanced presentation of a variety of approaches.

We would stress that our aim is not to support one model or another, but to offer a broad picture of work in progress. Throughout the book there is a lively sense of growth; no one is content to stand still, and everyone is committed to exploration, adaptation, and above all keeping an open mind, in the interests of improving patient and client care. We also hope that the contributions here will inspire you, if you are unfamiliar with the topic, to delve more deeply into the more extended work not just of our contributors but also of other nurses in the UK and abroad. The references and further reading lists should help you to trace the sources.

BETTY KERSHAW
JANE SALVAGE
November 1985

Introduction

Before you read the contributions it may be useful to look at nursing theories and nursing models as a whole and to consider how they relate to delivering nursing care using the problem-solving approach commonly referred to as the nursing process. There is currently much debate about the relationship between nursing models and nursing theories. Those who attended Discovery International's nurse theorist conference in Pittsburgh, USA, in May 1985 were able to listen to nurses presenting two sides of the argument: Roy and Orem postulated that nursing theories grew from clinical practice through analysing what nursing was and how nurses delivered care, while Rogers, Parse and King suggested that the theoretical framework was developed first, and that the guidelines for practice came out of the framework.

This book's purpose is not to present the case for or against the structural nature of a nursing theory. Here it suffices to say that, whether development commences at one end or the other, the nursing model interprets the theory for clinical practice, and it is to the model that nurse researchers, clinicians and educators look when seeking a basis for that practice.

Roy (1984) lists the essential elements of a model for nursing practice as:

a description of the person receiving care
a statement of the goal of nursing
a definition of health
a specified meaning of environment
a delineation of nursing activities

A model defines not only these concepts but also how they relate to one another. In this volume Chadderton gives an overview of Roy's own model which clearly illustrates how it incorporates all these essential elements. Castledine discusses the relationship between the Roy model and the nursing process, while Walsh conducts a similar exercise with Orem's model. The nursing process is emphatically not a model for nursing; it is one means of putting a model into practice, a tool or instrument and not a theory. If the chosen model contains all the essential elements of nursing, nurses using it as a framework for an individualised, problem-solving approach to care can be assured that it helps them to consider every single aspect of the nursing intervention needed by the patient.

Roper, Logan & Tierney focus on the patient's ability to perform activities of living. Thus the nurse carrying out the patient's initial interview will explore his or her ability to carry out these activities and assess the nursing needs. All the models explore the factors which affect the patient's ability to perform activities of living, and nursing action is then planned as appropriate; a nurse using the Roper, Logan & Tierney model would need to consider such factors as the patient's age (lifespan), living environment and socioeconomic status. Roy, too, sees the need for patient assessment to take into account their point on the 'life continuum', and as well as conducting a full physical assessment, the nurse must consider the patient's role function and dependency networks; consideration of the patient's developmental stage is indeed common to almost all models. Orem (1980) recognised that people's ability to care for themselves is directly related to their developmental stage in the life cycle. Like Roper et al, her model suggests that people's ability to care for themselves (or to carry out activities of living) is affected by environment and socialisation.

When considering the use of models in clinical practice, nurses often wonder whether they need to use only one, or whether several can be adapted for their specific use. This question was debated by the nurse theorists in Pittsburgh and they, like most British nurses, reached no firm conclusion. However, it was stressed that a model in its entirety should contain all the essential elements relating to care planning, and that those seeking to amalgamate models or to build their own needed to ensure that the framework presented a total perspective.

Both approaches have been adopted in the contributions to this book. Pearson describes the work of his unit based on one particular model – in this case that of Roper, Logan & Tierney – and highlights the neglected area of the role of the nurse using a model in relation to the multidisciplinary health care team. Castledine discusses how he has modified Roy's approach, while Chadderton has used Roy's model with little change.

Wright outlines his strong reservations about the blanket application of any particular model, and has taken positive steps to build one which he and his staff see as especially suitable for their patients. He stresses that any nursing model needs to be dynamic and fluid, and to develop as the practitioners learn from the experience of using it. Roy (1984) and Roper et al (1985) have documented how their models have changed over the years.

Wright also criticises the idea that any one model may be appropriate to every area of care. American hospitals will frequently integrate one particular nursing theory into their philosophy, thus directing the model of care to be used in the clinical units. This has implications for those managing the nursing service; here Farmer explores the role of management in the delivery of care using a nursing model, and says 'the reponsibility of the nurse manager for setting and monitoring standards requires the adoption of a model for nursing which reflects the values underlying the provision of services'. Yet in delineating the middle manager as an appropriate person to be involved in this, Farmer implicitly supports Pearson in allowing the clinical manager of each unit to select the most appropriate model.

Integral to working with models is the need to educate nurses in their use. Schools in America associated with a particular hospital may well build their curriculum on the model which that hospital uses; indeed, they may share a common philosophy. Nursing practice will be taught within the theoretical framework of the model, and alternative models will only be introduced late in the educative process. In the UK, too, it is becoming increasingly common for schools of nursing to follow the lead given by the universities and polytechnics and base their curriculum development on a nursing model. Vaughan helps to clarify many of the problems by identifying three possible approaches. Although she recognises that the single-model approach is easiest for the curriculum planner, she also describes a modular design in which appropriate models can be used when planning to meet teaching and learning needs in discrete areas. Thus the planner may use a specific model such as Neuman's – which stimulated Clark's development of a model for health visiting – or may explore the application of several models to a particular field, as Collister does here in his paper on psychiatric nursing.

Whichever model is chosen, however, it should be applied using the steps of the nursing process (Castledine's chapter includes guidelines for doing this, and should prove helpful to those beginning at the beginning). There are aspects of using this approach to care which need attention, though, in terms of broader societal issues and the availability of resources for health care. Does the use of a model imply a purely individualistic kind of care, with the nurse-patient relationship strictly one-to-one, or does it contain the potential for tackling the wider social dimension implied in much current thinking on health, as Clark implies? The nurse who assesses a patient using a model constructs a profile which may well raise issues around the patient's health and life about which she can do little. An unhappy relationship, unemployment or poor housing may all have significant effects on the patient's mental and physical well-being, for example. Walsh's critique of Orem's model on these lines points to a dimension of model use which needs further exploration.

Menzies (1961) noted that task allocation, the giving of care by rote, prevented the nurse from becoming closely involved with the patient. Using the nursing process based on a model makes it difficult for the nurse to avoid such intimacy, and there is evidence that nurses become stressed when they cannot cope with the strong feelings this may provoke in both nurse and patient. Gott (1983) also noted the stressful outcome when nurses were unable to assist patients to solve a problem which had been mutually identified. The use of models may well require much greater attention being paid to the nurse's welfare and the support she needs to carry out a demanding care programme – not only in terms of staffing levels, but in terms of her own psychological needs.

In the current political climate, resources for supporting the carers and for the delivery of care cannot keep pace with growing needs, to the detriment of care-giver and patient alike (Royal College of Nursing 1984). Nurses are increasingly documenting patient problems about which they can do little, or identifying nursing needs which cannot be met. On one hand the use of nursing models and the nursing process is being encouraged and there is no doubt, as Castledine, Pearson and Wright demonstrate, that once nurses are familiar with problem-solving it makes their care more effective and efficient. But if the planned care cannot be given because of financial constraints, perhaps it is realistic (and not defeatist) to emphasise that assessment should be directed solely and specifically to those patient needs which the nurse is able to meet through a constructive and achievable plan of care. In this light, the tale about the nurse who busily questioned her patient about his socioeconomic status, and whether his cat was being fed, while he was having a heart attack appears not just as a joke, but as a pertinent comment on the dangers of failing to use models as guidelines rather than as gospel.

On the positive side, the present emphasis on achieving value for money, and on the expectation that practitioners such as nurses and doctors should be able to demonstrate the benefits of their interventions through various types of audit, points to the need for nurses to develop tools to measure the standard of their care. Measurement, of course, is not simply a quantitative or financial issue, but we surely have a responsibility to the patients who place themselves in our trust to ensure that our work is effective and efficient as well as compassionate and committed. Increasingly, nurses are being obliged to prove to the non-nurses who hold the purse-strings precisely how their requests for better staffing levels and other resources can be justified. Basing nursing on a theoretical framework supported by research findings, and devising methods of using this approach to monitor the quality of care, could be a crucial weapon in the financial argument.

Finally – a point made explicitly or implicitly by all our contributors – the thinking and action stimulated by nursing models is helping nurses attack the long-neglected task of defining what nursing is and what knowledge, skills and attitudes are needed to do it. For too long we have floundered in a subordinate role, failing to identify the particular contribution nurses make to health care, picking up scraps of information or expertise from other disciplines without integrating them into a nursing framework. Now, however, we have the makings of a clear philosophy of nursing to underpin and shape our practice, management, education and research. It is our sincere hope that all those concerned about the quality of care – and we believe this means nearly all nurses – will find material in this collection to help them formulate their own philosophy and contribute to this vital debate.

References

Roy C (1984) *Introduction to Nursing: An Adaptation Model.* Englewood Cliffs NJ: Prentice-Hall

Orem D (1980) *Nursing: Concepts of Practice.* New York: McGraw-Hill

Roper N, Logan W & Tierney A (1985) *The Elements of Nursing.* Edinburgh: Churchill Livingstone

Menzies I (1960) *A Case Study in the Functioning of a Social System as a Defence against Anxiety.* London: Tavistock

Gott M (1983) In Davis B (ed) *Research into Nurse Education.* London: Croom Helm

Royal College of Nursing (1984) *Nurse Alert: A Report on the Effects of the Financial and Manpower Cuts in the NHS.* London: RCN

Models for Nursing
Edited by B Kershaw and J Salvage
© 1986 John Wiley & Sons Ltd.

1

The Value of Models for Care

JEAN McFARLANE

Why models?

Like most other occupational groups, nurses tend to pass through fashions in the way in which they carry out their work. There is a tendency to claim that team nursing, total patient care, holistic nursing, nursing process, accountability or management by objectives is the panacea for all the ills in nursing. The profession often divides into two camps – those who are 'in' on the latest thing and those who assiduously resist change. And now on top of the nursing process we have models!

It is a strange thing, too, that many of these ideas seem to come from people who have given up the practice of direct patient care – the educators, the managers, the statutory bodies and those people who generate syllabuses for university diplomas and degrees. Those who practise nursing for real are left to incorporate these new ideas into their practice with little help. They may even be denigrated for not changing their practice and so making it difficult for students to learn to nurse in the way they are being taught in the school. They landed the practitioners in the nursing process predicament, and now the models muddle.

The source of innovative ideas in nursing is in itself an interesting study. Nursing is a practice discipline and if its innovative ideas do not spring from practice then there will inevitably be an unreality about them and a lack of utility. By the same token, practice which is shorn of any theoretical basis and which does not allow its theoretical foundations to grow is not a practice discipline. It is a ritualised performance unrelated to the health care needs of individuals and society.

1

Thinking about nursing and changing practice is not easy. From analysis of the factors in a nursing situation and their relationship, a highly complex picture which emerges. At its simplest, two people interact to meet health care needs related particularly to daily living activities. The normal ability of one person to look after himself or herself (self care) may be impaired by disease or its treatment or by age, and physical, psychological, social and spiritual functioning is also involved. Meeting the needs may involve the use of complex scientific knowledge, technological applications and human relations skills. The context in which care is provided adds to the complexity, whether in the community or in an institution. No nursing situation is as simple as it looks, and intelligent decision-making and skilled performance in nursing are not easy.

In this complexity models may have a value for practice in a number of different ways. They may

   i   serve as a tool which links theory and practice;
   ii clarify our thinking about the elements of a practice situation and
       their relationship to each other;
   iii help practitioners of nursing to communicate with each other more
       meaningfully;
   iv serve as a guide to practice, education and research.

To justify these claims it is necessary, firstly, to look at the nature of models and their use, and some of the types of models of nursing which have been described. The rest of this book will present models as they have been used by nurses in the United Kingdom. You may then judge for yourself whether you find any of them a useful tool for practice.

The nature of models

Firstly, a warning! A great deal of the literature dealing with models is confusing, largely because the terminology is used inconsistently and the language is convoluted. Adam (1985), in a plea for greater clarity, gives examples of how inconsistently terms are used. This book is aimed primarily at nurses in the UK who come to the subject with little previous knowledge. Wider reading will reveal that the way in which terms are used may not always be consistent with the way in which they are used here. Perhaps we should issue a health warning – 'Reading this book and others in conjunction with it may cause mental indigestion'!

As I write I have a number of models around me – an inkstand with a model of a 1918 field ambulance on it, a doll dressed as a Welsh lady, a jade platypus from Australia, a reproduction of the first map of Wales printed in 1573, a black cat. My room is not inhabited by an ambulance, a Welsh lady, a platypus or the original map of Wales! A real black cat competes for space with the papers surrounding me, but he is a cat; the model is a representation of him, as are all the other models representations only of the reality that they represent.

Models of nursing, then, are representations of the reality of nursing practice. They represent the factors at work and how they are related. Part of their utility is that they make the factors in a nursing situation explicit. They become a tool which reminds us about different aspects of nursing care we may tend to ignore or forget. The fact that they portray relationships between factors is also useful. We are reminded of the relationship between physical and psychological factors and we take account of the relationship in giving nursing care. Of course, there are good and bad models. Sometimes in a gift shop we may be repelled by models which are a distortion of something that in reality is beautiful, like very crude flying ducks. We may also be overwhelmed with the ingenuity and detail of, say, a model ship in a bottle. Similarly, there are good and bad models of nursing. Some are crude and distort the reality of practice, some may get the relationships all wrong. A model developed by someone else in a different nursing situation and a different culture needs to be reviewed in our own practice situation – 'Is that how I see nursing?'. Better still, it is good to develop a model of our own and test it against others.

At one level, a model is a mental picture or private image of nursing practice, and we each have our own. In the field of sociology Inkeles (1966) said, 'Each sociologist carries in his head one or more models of society and man which greatly influence what he looks for, what he does with his observations by way of fitting them along with other facts into a larger scheme of explanation'. Moreover, 'every scientist has a general conception of the realm in which he is working – some mental picture of how it is put together and how it works'.

Most nurses have a rough picture of the general parameters of nursing which includes ideas about the nature and role of the patient or client and the nurse, the environment or culture in which nursing takes place, and the major field of nursing function, ie, health care and the nature of nursing methods or action. Flaskerud & Halloran (1980) summarise these as

> the person receiving the nursing;
> the environment within which the person exists;
> the health-illness continuum within which the person falls at the time of interaction with the nurse;
> nursing actions themselves.

Some authors represent these four central concepts as a model relating the concepts, others identify them as the paradigm of nursing (Thibodeau 1983), and still others the metaparadigm of nursing (Fawcett 1984). Without confusing ourselves with the differences in terminology at that level, the literature also refers to conceptual models and theoretical models (not to speak of conceptual frameworks and theoretical frameworks).

At a very simple level of definition, a conceptual model identifies and defines the factors or phenomena at work in a nursing situation and describes their relationship. A conceptual model is pretheoretical. A theoretical model, on the other hand, portrays the relationship of theories which have been tested empirically by research. The two kinds of models relate to different levels of theory development. Before nursing can develop theories on the basis of which practice can be prescribed, hypotheses about the relationship of concepts in nursing practice have to be formulated and tested and related to other available theories.

A conceptual model is derived largely from unsystematised empirical observations and induction, whereas a theoretical model is constructed from empirical research and established theories (Reilly 1975). The distinction, however, is unclear in the literature and when reading it is wise to question which type of model is being referred to.

A model is a conceptual tool and, like a tool, should be used appropriately and discarded or adapted for the needs of the job. It should not become a strait-jacket.

Types of models

Conceptual models can be categorised according to their primary focus. They represent different views and explanations about the nature of nursing goals, methods and the use of different theories about the person who is a patient.

Interaction models focus on the nature of nurse-patient interaction in nursing care and draw heavily on symbolic interactionism. Blumer (1969) originally outlined three essential premises of the theory.

(a)   'Human beings act towards things on the basis of the meanings that things have for them.'
(b)   'The meanings of such things is derived from or arises out of the social interaction that one has with one's fellows.'
(c)   'These meanings are handled in, and modified through, interpretive process used by the person in dealing with the things he encounters.'

It is understandable that psychiatric nurses have drawn heavily on interaction theory, but there is a growing recognition that nurse-patient interaction is fundamental in all fields of nursing and that finding meaning in a sickness situation is something to which the nurse contributes. Related concepts include communication, self-concept and role. Travelbee (1971), Riehl (1980), Orlando (1961) and King (1981) make use of interactionist models.

Developmental models focus on theories of development or change to explain the elements in a nursing situation. These include theories of physical, cognitive, social, spiritual and moral development through the life span. A developmental model is therefore extremely useful in the insights it provides into any aspect of nursing related to age (paediatric, geriatric nursing, and so on), but theorists like Peplau (1952) use developmental theory in describing the task of both nurse and patient finding personal development in a nursing situation. Thibodeau (1983) uses developmental theory to develop a 'crisis model' with three stages (pre-crisis, crisis and post-crisis). Developmental models represent the stage and direction of development, the form of development and potential for development in health situations.

Self-care, daily living, or activities of living or human needs models have a common basis of human needs for life and health as the focus of nursing action. Henderson (1966), Rogers (1970), Orem (1980) and Roper, Logan & Tierney (1980) fall into this category. Notably, Orem (1980) from her self-care model has generated and tested theories about self-care deficits, self care and dependant care and nursing systems.

Systems models make use of general systems theory as a basis for describing the elements of a nursing situation. The patient is regarded as an open system. Roy (1980) uses the physiological concept of adaptation within a systems framework. The system of the patient interacts with stressors in the environment and the nurse manipulates the patient system or the environment to aid adaptation in four modes. Johnson (1980) presents a behavioural systems model in which the patient is seen as a collection of behavioural subsystems. Neuman (1982) presents a health-care systems model in which the patient reacts to stressors at different levels of resistance and intervention is at the level of primary, secondary or tertiary prevention. Her model does not identify a unique nursing role – it is a multiprofessional model.

Although models may be categorised by their primary theoretical focus, most of them, in representing the complexity of nursing, include theoretical elements which predominate in others; interaction, development, self care, stress and adaptation occur in a great many. The mixed or eclectic model which makes use of more than one primary type of theory may well be more common than is thought.

Conflicts are inherent in the different theoretical stances taken in different models – some are mechanistic and some organismic in orientation. Some people would question whether a model which relies heavily on theories drawn from physiological functioning (stress adaptation) or social functioning (symbolic interaction) can wholly explain a nursing situation. Models using theories from nursing practice as an integrating theme are less common. In some so-called models the basis of nursing action is apparently omitted, and that is a significant omission. Can models which omit any one of the four elements in a nursing situation (the person nursed, the context of nursing, the health-illness situation and nursing action) in fact be true models of nursing?

Models in practice

The chapters which follow give examples of some of the different types of models as they have been used in the UK. In trying to evaluate them we need to review their possible usefulness in our own clinical practice.

It may be that none of the models presented here seems a comfortable 'fit' for your practice. Yet consciously or unconsciously we all use a model which guides our nursing goals and the methods of achieving them. Florence Nightingale's model of nursing was one in which the nurse controlled the environment to allow nature to cure the patient. Many nurses still see nursing as assisting the medical role and their model of nursing is a medical model, ie. the treatment of disease with the objective of cure. Some nurses' model of nursing is apparently a series of tasks related to body systems and their functions and the work of the organisation. But whatever model guides our nursing action, it indicates the kind of assessments we need to make, the goals of nursing care and how to achieve them. Conceptually it lies at the back of our thinking at each stage of the nursing process. It is a matter of some importance to make our personal model explicit, if only to ourselves.

References

Adam E (1985) Toward more clarity in terminology : frameworks, theories and models. *Journal of Nursing Education*, **24**(4), 151–155

Blumer H (1969) *Symbolic Interactionism: Perspective and Method*. New Jersey: Prentice Hall

Fawcett J (1984) *Analysis and Evaluation of Conceptual Models of Nursing*. Philadelphia: F A Davis

Flaskerud J H & Halloran E J (1980) Areas of agreement in nursing theory development. *Advances in Nursing Science*, **3**(1), 1–7

Henderson V (1966) *The Nature of Nursing*. New York: Macmillan

Inkeles A (1966) *What is Sociology?* New Jersey: Prentice Hall

Johnson D E (1980) In *Conceptual Models for Nursing Practice*. Norwalk, CT: Appleton-Century-Crofts

King I M (1981) *A Theory for Nursing : Systems Concept Process*. New York: John Wiley

Neuman B (1982) *The Neuman Systems Model : Application to Nursing Education and Practice*. Norwalk, CT: Appleton-Century-Crofts

Orem D (1980) *Nursing : Concepts of Practice*. New York: McGraw Hill

Orlando I J (1961) *The Dynamic Nurse – Patient Relationship : Function Process and Principles*. New York: Pitman

Peplau H (1952) *Interpersonal Relations in Nursing*. New York: Pitman USA

Reilly D (1975) Why a conceptual framework? *Nursing Outlook*, **23**(9). Referred to in Fawcett J The what of theory development. In NLN (1978) *Theory Development: Why, What, How?* Pub No 15 – 11708. New York: The League

Riehl J (1980) In Riehl J & Roy C (eds) (1980) *Conceptual Models for Nursing Practice*. Norwalk, CT: Appleton-Century-Crofts

Riehl J & Roy C (eds) (1980) *Conceptual Models for Nursing Practice*. Norwalk, CT: Appleton-Century-Crofts

Rogers M (1970) *An Introduction to the Theoretical Basis of Nursing*. Philadelphia: F A Davis

Roper N, Logan W W & Tierney A J (1980) *The Elements of Nursing*. Edinburgh: Churchill Livingstone

Roy C (1980) In Riehl J & Roy C (1980) *Conceptual Models for Nursing Practice*. Norwalk, CT: Appleton-Century-Crofts

Travelbee J (1971) *Interpersonal Aspects of Nursing*. Philadelphia: F A Davis

Thibodeau J A (1983) *Nursing Models: Analysis and Evaluation*. Monterey, Calif: Wadsworth Health Sciences Division

Models for Nursing
Edited by B Kershaw and J Salvage
©1986 John Wiley & Sons Ltd.

2
Exploring the Issues

ELIZABETH FARMER

Unprecedented social, scientific and technological changes have increased the complexity of caring and brought fresh challenges to those reponsible for the provision of health care. Escalating costs and uncertain outcomes of health services have prompted calls for ways of identifying needs and of determining how needs are best met. These concerns are set against a background of growing doubts about the wisdom of trying to develop services based on the highly abstract concepts of health and needs, and increasing criticism of the tendency to encompass all human problems under the umbrella of 'health'.

Amid the controversy about the 'roles' and 'goals' of health services the practice of nursing has been looked at critically, resulting in claims that nursing practice is based on inadequate problem definition, subjective recall of evidence and unsophisticated generalising. One response to the critics has been to intensify the development of models for nursing within which to identify more concrete, realistic goals for practice.

Historically the practice of nursing has taken place within a modified medical model which has a disease/treatment orientation. Nursing curricula and the patterns of organising and managing nursing resources have evolved from this model. Most of the nursing models which have been constructed as alternatives to the disease/treatment approach have been founded on 'human needs' perspectives (for example, Roy & Riehl 1974, and King 1971). Others have taken a 'functional' approach to the development of models for nursing (for example the Scottish National Nursing and Midwifery Consultative Committee, 1976; Roper, Logan & Tierney 1980).

In line with this the advantages of a systematic approach to nursing were increasingly being extolled. For example, 'it is through the systematic and scientific process that the discipline will be further developed, practice will be improved and patients will benefit' (WHO 1981). The underlying assumption is that through the use of a systematic problem-solving approach within a person-centred model, nursing practice is accurately informed, dynamic and objective rather than intuitive or tradition-bound. Nursing care is based on a critical analysis of patients' requirements for effective living, and their ability or otherwise to meet these requirements independently, rather than on speculation and assumption.

The development and use of person-centred models for nursing and of a systematic problem-solving method as the dynamic force which activates the model should emphasise the necessary and intimate relationship between nursing practice, research, education and management. Unfortunately this relationship has been obscured by misperceptions and misinterpretations about the role and function of models and a systematic approach to nursing. The consequences are briefly described below.

A systematic approach to nursing

The literature on the introduction of a systematic approach to nursing highlights an interactive and interchangeable use of the terms *nursing process*; *problem solving*; *scientific method*; and the *process of nursing*. For example, Marriner (1979) defines the nursing process as 'the application of scientific problem-solving to nursing care'. McFarlane & Castledine (1982) refer to it as 'a systematic method of decision-making and planning nursing care', while Roper *et al* describe the process of nursing as 'a process of problem-solving in a rational and scientific manner'. The Scottish National Nursing and Midwifery Consultative Committee holds that 'nursing is a process with definable phases which take place in specific situations requiring a greater or lesser degree of independent judgement'.

The variable use of terms has been misleading and has attracted criticism. On the other hand, it may be interpreted as part of a process of clarification of meaning as a consequence of experience and in response to criticism. Certainly the term *nursing process* has led to the incorrect belief that the logical problem-solving approach implicit in the term is unique to nursing, rather than being an adaptation from general use.

The more recent preference for the terms *the process of nursing* and *the systematic method* further indicates the desire for clarity of meaning, and particularly to distinguish between the content and the method of nursing. In response, Prophit (1980) among others has expressed the belief that the art and science of nursing have a symbiotic relationship. As she noted, 'without the art there is no reason for the science, and without the science, there are no data for the art'.

Furthermore, the emphasis on the method of nursing has led to the incorporation of the 'nursing process' in nursing curricula as an added extra rather than being central to nursing content. That this distinction between method and content has not been obvious may be explained, in part, by the tendency to give subtle clues in definitions and other writings rather than to make explicit the essential links. For example: '*scientific* problem-solving' (Marriner 1979); 'systematic method of *decision making*' (McFarlane & Castledine 1982);

'*independent judgement*' (SNNMCC 1976). As Prophit noted, 'whether one speaks of building science, problem-solving, nursing process, or research, the method is consistent; *underlying the method is the process of critical reflective thought*'.

Critical thinking involves the ability to recognise the existence of problems and acceptance of the need to suspend judgement until evidence has been gathered to confirm the presence and exact nature of the problem. In the process of critical thinking, past experiences and existing knowledge guide the search for evidence in support of assertions and determine the value which is attached to the various types of evidence.

Nursing developments – the need for direction

A change in the framework for nursing and, within this, the adoption of a systematic approach to nursing–implicit in which is the process of critical reflective thought–is believed to give a new perspective to the problems in nursing (Walter *et al* 1976), ultimately leading to an improvement in nursing care. It is assumed that this approach will unite practice, education, management and research in a joint effort to meet the changing needs for nursing care. New possibilities for solutions to apparently insoluble problems are revealed when the problems are viewed from a different standpoint. The hope, therefore, must be for evolutionary and co-ordinated change rather than revolutionary and fragmented change. As Watzlawick *et al* (1974) noted, 'history offers an embarrassingly long list of revolutions whose end results were, by and large, more of the same conditions which the revolution had set out to overthrow and replace by a brave new world'.

There is evidence of this phenomenon in numerous reports on the apparently persistent problems in nursing management and education, in which issues of 'roles', 'goals' and 'rewards' are addressed without regard for the underlying awareness that the 'pieces' of nursing do not fit together coherently in the medical model. Without a shared philosophy for nursing, there are likely to be further costly, piecemeal developments resulting in fragmented services, guaranteed to create divisions rather than unity because there is no master plan into which they can all fit comfortably. Also, without a master plan it will not be possible to discriminate between 'good' and 'bad' plans, creating a risk that the baby will be thrown out with the bath water.

The directive to nurses to become 'patient-centred' has raised issues concerning the effective deployment of resources. Consequently 'team nursing', 'patient allocation' and 'primary nursing' have been proposed as ways of providing individualised nursing care and of increasing job satisfaction while making more effective use of resources. Though the introduction of a systematic approach to nursing created an awareness of the need to improve, for example, communication and observation skills, there is little evidence to suggest that questions were simultaneously raised about the foundations of nursing practice. Experimenting with methods of managing nursing care without knowing what is to be managed is likely to produce confusion, discontent and rejection of potentially useful developments.

In recognition of the need for continuity of nursing care and therefore of the importance of documentation, much attention has been given to the development of nursing records systems. Unfortunately the structure of the nursing record has received more attention than its content. The possibilities for gathering information about nursing from nurses' records have been increased through computer technology, but the potential for development cannot be realised without a unifying framework for nursing within which appropriate questions may be posed and answers considered.

Similarly, the systematic documentation of nursing (implicit in the systematic approach to nursing) revealed possibilities for measuring the quality of nursing care. There has been an upsurge of interest in quality assurance programmes, notably those developed by Phaneuf (1976) and Hegyvary & Haussman (1975). Related to this is the work of the Royal College of Nursing (1981) on the definition of standards of nursing care.

All these activities have been constrained by the lack of agreement on what constitutes good nursing care and, most particularly and fundamentally, on how to choose a framework for nursing within which to address the issues. McFarlane (1976), among others, has noted that the differences between the frameworks offered may be concerned more with emphasis than substance; there is something to be gained from the adoption of any of the frameworks because they describe and inform nursing more accurately than the existing medical model.

Learning from experience

Tobin et al (1979) argued that 'the effectiveness of nursing personnel in carrying out their assigned duties depends on the interdependence between the administrative and educational functions exercised by the nursing organization.' If there is no agreement on what is expected and how well it is to be done, 'there can be little agreement in the identification of discrepancies that indicate learning needs or in the subsequent programming necessary to develop the personnel.'

For nurse educators, the challenge of patient-centred nursing derives from propositions about the ways in which knowledge is gained and used, and, relative to this, about the methods of learning.

The role of experience in learning (Knowles 1970) and in motivating towards continuing learning (Copp 1975) has been increasingly emphasised in the literature on education in general, and in nursing in particular. Here the assertion that work and learning should be integrated (Roper 1976) seems valid. Indeed, the belief that the 'theory' and practice of nursing should be closely linked was supported through the introduction in Scotland of a modular system of education which aims to provide learning experiences which have sequence, continuity and unity. This development is essentially of a structural rather than a substantive nature. The framework for nursing focuses observations and helps to order experiences and inform action; if the content of the nursing curriculum remains the same (in the face of assertions that it is inappropriate), reshuffling the work experiences will not necessarily make them more relevant or meaningful.

According to Schoen (1979), 'nurses who are effective practitioners invariably continue to learn on the job, but too often this is incidental, rather than planned learning.' Postbasic education in nursing has been fragmented and geared largely to the acquisition of specialist skills in response to scientific and technological developments. In the absence of a unifying framework for nursing within which to locate the focus of new skills and knowledge, postbasic courses will continue to produce specialist groups of nurses with ambiguous roles.

Planned change in nursing

Continuing or lifelong learning was viewed by Toffler (1970) as affording protection against the adverse effects of change. He held that 'by introducing change, wherever possible, in the form of predictable rather than erratic chains of events, we can help provide elements of continuity even in the midst of social upheaval'.

Change happens when one or more people perceive that a problem exists and that change is desirable and possible. The need to plan change and the role of education in effecting change is increasingly acknowledged. If it is accepted that adults are motivated to learn through encountering problems in their immediate situation, then the link between planned change and education becomes more apparent. It is, however, necessary to have a model within which to identify the need for change and to plan and evaluate the change. Action research is regarded as the vehicle for change (Chin & Benne 1976). There is also increasing support for the role of action research in promoting the growth and development of nursing knowledge.

Building knowledge through practice

According to Chinn & Jacobs (1978), 'what has not been accomplished in most thinking and problem solving is the critical analysis of ideas, their systematic organisation into relational statements and their validation in empirical reality'. It has been suggested that nurse practitioners hold a key position in knowledge-building and testing propositions (Shröck 1981), yet practising nurses appear to have difficulty in seeing themselves as researchers. Basic nurse education does not promote or develop critical thinking, which is one of the common links between nursing practice, research, education and management. Moreover the types of problem which designated nurse researchers have so far chosen to investigate, and the sophisticated methods used to study particular problems, create an impression of research as an élitist activity. Finally, some research findings have no immediate usefulness, or have tenuous links with practice.

The divide between research and practice could be narrowed through the use of models for nursing as a means of identifying and addressing more concrete and immediate nursing problems. Nurses might also have less difficulty accepting research as part of their role if action research were promoted and attempts made to emphasise the similarities between action research and the systematic problem-solving approach which is the process part of nursing. Isaac & Michael (1971) have stated that the purpose of action research is to develop new skills or new approaches, and to solve problems with direct application to the classroom or working world setting. Table 2.1 compares the steps in action research and a systematic problem-solving method. One of their common properties is critical reflective thought. Another is that they are both dynamic processes operating feedback mechanisms in response to the ongoing situation.

Table 2.1

Steps in Action Research		Systematic Problem-Solving Method	
1	Define the problem	1	Recognition of the problem
2	Review the literature (to specify precisely the problem and guide investigation)	2	Collect information (to specify precisely the problem and guide care planning)
3	Set objectives	3	Set objectives (within which are the evaluation criteria)
4	Select approaches and procedures to meet objectives	4	Consider possible solutions to the problem
5	Establish evaluation criteria	5	Select appropriate solution
6	Analyse the data and evaluate the outcomes	6	Carry out the plan
		7	Evaluate the outcomes

Action research can be used by nurses to guide, correct and evaluate decisions and actions concerned with resolving problems. The information gathered in particular situations can be used to guide actions in similar situations in the future. In this regard action research has knowledge-building potential; as well as being of practical use in the immediate sense, it has value as an exploratory tool for highlighting areas requiring more study.

Parallels can be drawn between the knowledge-building potential of action research and the possibilities of development through the documentation of nursing implicit in the nursing process. The documentation of care and the evaluation of outcomes gives nurses opportunities to identify their own learning needs. Self-motivated learning would be an expected outcome of the critical analysis of nursing care planning. Similarly, the exploration of nurses' values and their relationship to priorities for nursing care, and the expected outcomes of care, is more likely through the systematic provision and evaluation of nursing care than with traditional task-oriented, intuitive forms of nursing.

Nursing practice, research, education and management are interdependent and are linked through the use of a systematic method within a model for nursing. These points are reinforced in the practical example below, which is drawn from my experience of providing nursing services for the elderly.

Using models for the provision of nursing services

The 1981 report on nursing line management in the National Health Service states that 'middle management exists to facilitate the delivery of the nursing services. Its unique role lies in appointing appropriately qualified staff, planning continuing education, setting and monitoring standards, and involvement in all aspects concerned with making the most effective use of resources'. The responsibility of the nurse manager for setting and monitoring standards requires the adoption of a model for nursing which reflects the values underlying the provision of services. Hirschfeld (1981) holds that 'respect for persons is the ethical base for search of knowledge and provision of services for the elderly'. If this view is supported, the model for nursing should reflect person-centredness. In addition to an appropriate model, a method of evaluating service provision will be necessary.

Donabedian (1966) advocated the use of a systematic method for evaluating medical care and suggested that the factors influencing care might be classified as *structure*, *process*, and *outcome*. Structure is concerned with environmental factors such as architecture; administrative arrangements; volume of work; manpower and goals of the organisation. Process refers to the skills, knowledge and attitudes of the people working in the structure. Outcome is the consequence of the interaction of the structure and process elements. A systematic method, in the form of action research, is used in association with the chosen model for nursing and the framework for evaluation to address the problems affecting the provision of nursing services.

The problem I have chosen to illustrate the practical value of models concerns a persistent shortage of patients' underwear. On closer examination, three groups of factors contributed to the problem: The use of heat-sealed identification labels which became unstuck or shrivelled up during laundering causing the garments to tear; a directive favouring thermochemical treatment which meant all underwear was sent to other hospitals for laundering; a resulting shortage compounded by the failure to take into account the needs of patients as individuals when calculating requirements.

The review of relevant literature was guided by Orem's (1980) self-care concepts of nursing, and focused particularly on the provision of personal clothing services for the elderly; methods of identifying individual patients' clothing, taking account of the need for comfort and dignity; and the arguments for and against thermochemical treatment of underwear.

The objectives established following this review were that there should be adequate supplies of underwear to suit individual needs and preferences; the system of laundering should be bacteriologically safe; there should be no loss of garments through faults in laundering; the systems of laundering and labelling should be cost-effective; and the system of labelling should be permanent, permit easy identification of personal clothing, and provide comfort for and preserve the dignity of patients. The measures taken to meet the objectives are organised under the structure and process components of the framework for evaluation.

Structure

(i)   An inventory of patients' personal clothing, including the items in the laundry system.

(ii) Examining the claims concerning the usefulness of various types of labels.

(iii) Examining the practical and financial implications of laundering the

underwear in the hospital.
(iv)   Comparing the costs of labelling systems.

Process

(i)   Monitoring incontinence levels.
(ii)   Examining procedures for separating and despatching soiled garments to the laundry.
(iii)   Carrying out bacteriological monitoring of underwear in a trial in the personal clothing laundry.

As a result, more garments were bought to meet individual needs. Reusable individual name tapes were introduced and arrangements were made for most underwear to be laundered in the hospital. So all the objectives were met. As well as the improvement in patient services, there were gains in knowledge of the organisation and management of patient services and for the development of nursing. In particular, it was shown that there was a need to work towards a shared philosophy for care among the staff groups, so that quality and cost-effectiveness might co-exist. There was justification for questioning disinfection policies which could be counter-productive in some instances. In this way, nurse practitioners had an opportunity to contribute to policy-making. Finally, the problem of the underwear initiated a critical examination of nursing practices concerned with the management of incontinence.

The aim of this essay was to create an awareness of the interdependence of nursing practice, research, education and management through the use of a systematic method within an appropriate model for nursing. Individual nurses have different values, beliefs and talents which create preferences for certain activities and experiences and so make us essentially practitioners, researchers, educators or managers. Whatever our preferences, there is a shared knowledge-base and a common core of skills in nursing; the differences lie in the depth of knowledge needed in certain situations and in the predominance of particular groups of skills. Persistent attempts to create unnatural divisions may hinder rather than help the development of nursing.

Acknowledgement

Much of the material in this chapter was drawn from a review of the literature contained in a report* prepared by the author for the Scottish Home and Health Department Health Services Research Committee, who also funded the original work. The views contained in the report are not necessarily supported by the Committee.

---

*Farmer, E S (1985) *On Introducing a Systematic Method for the Practice and Study of Nursing*. Edinburgh: Nursing Research Unit, University of Edinburgh

References

Chin R & Benne K D (1976) General strategies for effecting changes in human systems. In Bennis *et al* (eds) *The Planning of Change*. New York: Holt, Rinehart & Winston

Chinn P & Jacobs M (1978) A model for theory development in nursing. *Advances in Nursing Science*, **1**(1), 1–11

Copp L A (1975) Inservice education copes with resistance to change. *Journal of Continuing Education in Nursing*, **6**(2), 19–27

Donabedian A (1966) *Evaluating the Quality of Medical Care*. Millbank Mem. Fund, Q.44, (Part 2). July, 166–206

Hegyvary S T & Haussman R K D (1975) Monitoring nursing care quality. *Journal of Nursing Administration*, **5**(5), 17–26

Hirschfeld M J (1979) Research in nursing gerontology. *Journal of Advanced Nursing*, **4**, 622

Isaac S & Michael W B (1971) *Handbook in Research and Evaluation*. San Diego, California: Edits Publishers

King I M (1971) *Toward a Theory for Nursing*. New York: J Wiley & Sons

Knowles M S (1970) *The Modern Practice of Adult Education*. New York: Association Press

Marriner A (1979) *The Nursing Process*. St. Louis: C V Mosby Co

McFarlane J K (1976) The role of research and the development of nursing theory. *Journal of Advanced Nursing*, **1**, 443–451

McFarlane J K & Castledine G (1982) *A Guide to the Practice of Nursing Using the Nursing Process*. London: The C V Mosby Company

Orem D E (1980) *Nursing: Concepts of Practice*. New York: McGraw-Hill

Phaneuf M C (1976) *The Nursing Audit: Self-regulation in Nursing Practice*. New York: Appleton-Century-Crofts

Prophit P (ed) (1980) *Documentation of the Nursing Process: The Reasons for Records*. Working Group on the Documentation of the Nursing Process, Bern, 8–12 December. Copenhagen: WHO

Roper N, Logan W W & Tierney A J (1980) *The Elements of Nursing*. Edinburgh: Churchill Livingstone

Roper N (1976) *Clinical Experience in Nurse Education*. Edinburgh: Churchill Livingstone

Roy C L & Riehl J P (1974) *Conceptual Models for Nursing Practice*. New York: Appleton-Century-Crofts

Royal College of Nursing (1981) *Towards Standards: A Discussion Document*. Second Report of the RCN Working Committee on Standards of Nursing Care (England and Wales). London: RCN

Schoen D E (1979) Lifelong learning: How some participants see it. *Journal of Continuing Education in Nursing*, **10**(2), 3–16

Scottish National Nursing and Midwifery Consultative Committee (1976) A new concept of nursing. Occasional Paper, *Nursing Times*, 8 April, 49–52

Schröck R A (1981) Philosophical issues. In Hockey L (ed) *Current Issues in Nursing*. Edinburgh: Churchill Livingstone

SHHD (1981) *Nursing Line Management in the National Health Service in*

Scotland. Edinburgh: SHHD

Tobin H M, Yoder Wise P S & Hull P K (1979) *The Process of Staff Development: Components for Change*. St. Louis: C V Mosby Co

Toffler A (1970) *Future Shock*. New York: Random House

Walter J B, Pardee G P & Molbo D M (1976) *Dynamics of Problem-Oriented Approaches: Patient Care and Documentation*. Philadelphia: J B Lippincott Company

Watzlawick P, Weakland J & Fisch R (1974) *Change: Principles of Problem Formation and Problem Resolution*. New York: W W Norton & Company

WHO (1981) *Proposal for a Study of Needs for Nursing Care, Planning, Implementation and Evaluation of Care Provided by Nurses Using Two Selected Groups of People in the European Region*. ICP/PPM 002, January. Copenhagen: WHO.

Models for Nursing
Edited by B Kershaw and J Salvage
© 1986 John Wiley & Sons Ltd.

3

Models in
Curriculum Development

BARBARA VAUGHAN

The purpose of this paper is to explore the implications of the current interest in nursing models from an educational stance, and to consider some of the issues that it raises for nurse educators, particularly in relationship to curriculum development. There is no doubt that there are dilemmas to be faced and that the answers are not clear-cut. But alternative approaches must be recognised and analysed before a considered choice can be made.

Three approaches to the use of a nursing model in curriculum design are outlined. No answers are offered since the final choice of approach must be made from within each individual educational institution. However, the reality of the difficulty faced by those nurses concerned with curriculum design is discussed, alongside the advantages and disadvantages of the choices available.

It is difficult to argue with the view that the first step in developing a curriculum for a practice discipline such as nursing is to identify the underlying conceptual framework. That framework will contain the theories and concepts which will go towards building the curriculum, and in turn the theories and concepts will reflect the beliefs and values of the discipline concerned, as well as the desired behaviour of the 'end product' of the programme, whether that is a nurse, a teacher or someone in another occupational group. The question to be raised is from where the starting point of such a framework should come. Should nurse educators be influential in directing practice, as has been the traditional pattern in nursing, or should it be practice that influences education? While some may argue otherwise, there is no doubt in my mind that at least the starting point must come from practice. While nurse educators are very well placed to refine and develop theories, both 'of' practice and 'for' practice, it does not seem appropriate that they are the ones actually to direct practice. Not only does it seem inappropriate, but there is also a fear that it will be ineffective.

We are already aware of the gap between theory and practice, the so-called

17

real-ideal gap, where what is taught is not what is seen in practice. Ways of minimising and not accentuating this dilemma must be sought. The risk of creating 'reality shock' (Kramer 1974), a reaction to the difference between how you believe things should be and how they really are, is very real for neophyte nurses, particularly as there is a movement away from the current apprenticeship-type approach to a more controlled way of managing nurse education. Curricula designed apart from the reality of what is seen in practice can only worsen this.

So the major dilemma that nurse educators face is that they need, or indeed must have a conceptual framework from which to develop the curriculum. But if that framework does not match practice they are at risk of exaggerating the real-ideal gap between theory and practice and moving from reality stress, already present, to reality shock. If they choose a nursing model from which to develop the curriculum in isolation, without exploring the feelings of practice, the danger is very real.

The crucial factor that the nursing model used in practice should reflect the personal views of the team concerned has been raised elsewhere, with emphasis laid on the team's right to choose for themselves. While theories and concepts can be taught, unless nurses actually believe in them they are unreal and their influence on practice will be lost. So the second major question is 'Can we expect all nursing units within a clinical district to base their practice on a single model?' If this expectation is real, who should make the choice? And if it is unreal, what are the implications for nurse educators in relationship to curriculum design?

Current approaches

Currently, two different approaches can be identified. One takes a specific model from which the curriculum is designed; the other finds a starting point in a particular clinical setting.

Firstly, some educational institutes have adopted a specific model for practice from which they have designed the curriculum. The model gives direction to

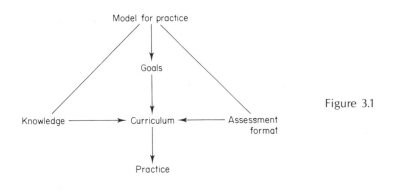

Figure 3.1

the knowledge required, the goals of practice advocated, and, among other things, the information gathered during assessment, all of which are incorporated into the curriculum. But what happens in practice if there is no match?

Student nurses at present move rapidly from one clinical area to another and are exposed to a wide variety of approaches to practice. In order to achieve a match between the curriculum model and the practice model, it would be necessary for all the clinical nurses working in areas where students are present to use a common approach which reflects the curriculum. Yet if there is a belief that the choice of model should arise from practice, and that different clinical areas may choose different approaches, then there is an obvious difficulty. It is the practitioners with students under their supervision who are faced with the dilemma. Do they try and adjust their practice in order that it should reflect the curriculum model? Or do they try and cope with the inevitable problem of having a rapid succession of students moving through their units, all of whom are familiar with a different framework for assessment and possibly with beliefs about the broad goals of practice which vary from those actually in use? (Figure 3.1). Some institutes in the USA have taken this approach, requiring that all clinical units follow the same model for practice and arguing that it is the most suitable way forward to develop the curriculum fully. Yet if there is a fundamental belief in the right of clinical teams to choose the model on which they base their practice, such a stance raises major difficulties.

An alternative approach tried in the UK has been to find a starting point in one particular clinical unit (see Wright's chapter in this volume). The ideas, beliefs and values of that team of nurses are explored and made explicit. They are then compared with existing well-developed models and a match sought. With a little bit of give and take on both sides, some adjustments to the views of the people concerned and some adjustments to the model, the result can be a clearly-defined nursing model based on a well-documented nursing framework. From this point on the development of the curriculum is relatively straightforward, although still an arduous task like any curriculum work (Figure 3.2).

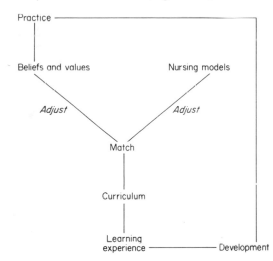

Figure 3.2

These first steps can only be commended, but there are still problems in the further outcomes. The curriculum will have been based on the views, beliefs and practice of one particular clinical unit. Yet, as we are all aware, one of the attractions of nursing is its very diversity. If the unit of learning concerned with the initial clinical setting is based on experience from that setting then all is well. The difficulty arises when it is transferred to a unit of learning concerned with a completely different clinical experience, where the model of practice may be quite different. For example, a group of nurses working in the community may choose to base their practice on a self-care framework, while those working in an acute surgical unit may find that a stress adaptation model reflects their views more accurately. Thus, if the whole curriculum is based on the model of those nurses working in the first unit, there is likely to be a discrepancy between theory and practice when the students move to work in the second unit. To obtain a match and to avoid the potential anguish of such a situation, the very fact that a difficulty exists must be acknowledged and handled in the teaching programme (Figure 3.3).

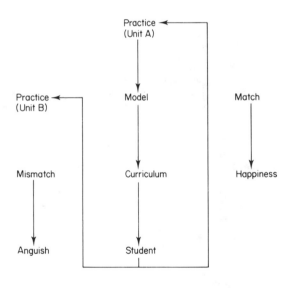

Figure 3.3

Alternative approaches

Having highlighted some of the very real difficulties that nurse educators face ·today, it is also necessary to consider some solutions and their advantages and disadvantages. Each solution offered is a viable proposition, but their difficulties must be recognised and coping mechanisms incorporated in the programme.

The eclectic approach

In this approach, thoughts and ideas from several well-documented models are amalgamated to form a very broad-based curriculum; in other words an attempt is made to create a new unified model incorporating many different concepts. But there is a danger that what is gained in breadth may be lost in depth. Models for practice not only contain clearly defined theories and concepts, they also consider their relationship and their application to nursing practice. In using ideas from many different models there is a risk that the network of ideas which links them together may be lost. It is not an impossible task, and indeed this is how models for practice have been developed, but it is protracted and difficult. Without such background work the framework on which the curriculum is built may be weak, and rather than leading to an integrated approach it may result in the presentation of fragmented and unrelated material.

It is always exciting to see the development of new ideas and the way in which they relate to nursing practice, but the enormity of the task must be recognised. In such an approach it is essential not only to identify the underlying beliefs, values, goals and knowledge but also their relationship to each other and to practice.

The single model approach

Here a single well-developed model is chosen from which the curriculum is developed. From the curriculum stance there is no doubt that this is the ideal solution, since the components which go towards curriculum design can all be found in any well-described practice model. They describe the underlying value system, the desired goals of practice and the knowledge considered essential for practice.

The dangers of this approach have already been discussed—the variance between what is taught and what is seen in practice and the resultant reality shock. Yet there are ways of overcoming such difficulties. Close links and the provision of continuing education for practising nurses can lead to an alteration in practice itself and a united approach in learning environments. Practising nurses' understanding of the curriculum model can lead to a deeper perception of the difficulties faced by students. Sessions can be incorporated in the learning programme to ensure that students are aware of the diversity of approaches they will find in their clinical experience. But if this overall method is adopted, the difficulties experienced by both clinical nurses and students must be made explicit if they are to be handled effectively.

A further word of caution about this approach: students who only have the opportunity to see nursing from a single model approach may potentially narrow their own sights. There are such diverse ways in which nursing care can be offered that it would seem rather sad not to offer them at least an insight into various different models for practice at an early stage in their nursing career, and help them to develop the critical skills they need to choose the right approach for themselves.

A modular approach

A third approach that could be taken is to follow a modular design. Here the curriculum is divided into discrete areas identified around nursing needs, for example long stay needs in institutions; acute episodic illness; primary care or care of the elderly. Unity would be sought in each area of practice and the curriculum designed around the appropriate model. Thus year one of training may deal with primary care, and both practice and the curriculum may reflect a developmental model. In the second year nursing needs relating to episodic illness may be covered using an adaptation model, and in year three looking at the special needs of the elderly an interactionist model may be employed. The timespan and relationship of particular models to particular areas of practice is arbitrary and would depend on the nature of the programme.

In this way, not only would students avoid the dilemma of the model for practice varying from the curriculum model, but they would also be exposed to a diversity of approaches. They would have the opportunity to analyse various models and compare their use in practice. The difficulties of moving to work in a different district after qualifying and having to learn a different framework would largely be overcome.

However, as in all situations there are disadvantages too. The complexity of the curriculum design would be great and the length of time taken to understand the differing concepts would have to be considered. There would have to be flexibility in teaching as changes occurred in practice, and the links between the two areas would have to be very close. Nevertheless it is an approach which must be considered.

There are doubtless other approaches to curriculum design relating to linking theory with the reality of practice and identifying the model of nursing to be used. The three above approaches have been outlined mainly as a way of demonstrating the dilemma that has to be faced by nurse educators. No attempt has been made to suggest which is the 'best' way, since there is no right or wrong answer and each approach has advantages and disadvantages. Provided the strengths and weaknesses are recognised and accounted for in the programme, the final choice must lie with the individual groups of people concerned. Indeed, there would be value in adopting a number of different approaches and evaluating the outcome in terms of the performance of the qualified nurses.

However, the argument may be related to an even more fundamental difficulty in the current nursing structure. While education and practice remain as two related but separate paths, the difficulty of linking theory with practice is unlikely to be overcome. If a way forward could be found to develop teacher practitioner roles, with a responsibility for teaching being combined with the authority for practice, some of the difficulties might be overcome—although recognition of the added responsibilities in such a role would have to be reflected in better staffing levels. Theoretical aspects of the course and clinical experience could then be closely linked with much greater ease. The current interest in joint appointments goes some way towards a solution, but is only a beginning to exploring the development of roles. Perhaps it is the major challenge for the future in resolving some of the dilemmas currently being faced in curriculum design.

Further Reading

Bevais E O (1978) *Curriculum Building in Nursing.* St Louis: C V Mosby Co

De Back V (1981) The relationship between senior nursing students ability for forming nursing diagnoses and a curriculum model. *Advances in Nursing Science,* **3**(3), 51–66

Clark J (1982) Development of models and theories on the concept of nursing. *Journal of Advanced Nursing,* **7,** 129–134

Fawcett J (1984) *Analysis and Evaluation of Conceptual Models of Nursing.* Philadelphia: F A Davies

Kramer M (1974) *Reality Shock: Why Nurses Leave Nursing.* St Louis: C V Mosby Co

Pearson A (1983) *The Clinical Nursing Unit.* London: Heinemann

Pearson A & Vaughan B (1986) *Nursing Models in Practice.* London: Heinemann

Pietroni P (1984) Holistic medicine – new map, old territory. *British Journal of Holistic Medicine,* **1,** 3–13

Torres G & Yura H (1973) *Today's Conceptual Framework: Its Relationship to the Curriculum Development Process.* No 15–1529. National League for Nursing, Publ 1–12: New York

4

Nursing Models: A Process of Construction and Refinement

NANCY ROPER
WINIFRED LOGAN
ALISON TIERNEY

> 'Thus the task is, not so much to see what no one has seen yet; but to think what nobody has thought yet, about what everybody sees.'–SCHOPENHAUER

All nurses, of course, assume that they *know* what 'nursing' is! Why then has the question 'What is nursing?' continued to tax the minds of nurses over the years? Are we now any nearer to making explicit our understanding of the nature of nursing? Recall the words of Florence Nightingale (1859): 'It has been said and written scores of times that every woman makes a good nurse. I believe on the contrary that the very elements of nursing are all but unknown'. To a great extent the challenge of that statement still remains.

However, in recent years, it seems as if the challenge has been taken up with considerable vigour and determination. Although this is as evident in the UK as in any part of the world, British nurses have not written much about their scholarly endeavours until relatively recently. In contrast North American nurses have been publishing theoretical and epistemological papers for some 30 years. Among the frontrunners, in the 1950s, came Hildegarde Peplau, Virginia Henderson, Dorothy Johnson and Lydia Hall; more recently, names such as Martha Rogers, Callista Roy, Dorothea Orem and Betty Neuman lengthen the roll of American nurse theorists. Each has made a particular contribution in her own right, but what they have done collectively is to encourage nurses in the pursuit of theory development in nursing. It is both fascinating and enlightening to trace the unfolding of this development in the USA over the past three decades, and a masterly review and analysis is provided in a recently published text by Meleis (1985). Commenting on the present, Meleis says, 'The 1980s are characterized by an acceptance of the significance of theory for nursing and, furthermore, by the inevitability of the need for the development of nursing theory.'

Are we, here in the UK, at such a stage? Probably it is unrealistic to claim an overall 'acceptance' of nursing theory, but what is evident is an ever-increasing *awareness* and, without any doubt, a high level of interest. This interest is not confined to the groves of academe–witness the response from a broad cross-section of the nursing community to the *Senior Nurse* Manchester conference on which the idea and substance of this book is based. It might be speculated that, when an historical analysis is published in years to come, the 1980s almost certainly will be viewed as the threshold of an era of theory development in British nursing.

It is interesting to ponder what place in that history will be accorded to the Roper, Logan & Tierney model for nursing. A model is, of course, only an intermediate stage in theory development; and this particular model will take its place alongside others which have been developed or adapted for use by nurses in the UK. One interesting thing will be to see the date attached to the Roper, Logan & Tierney model for nursing.

The model, as it is now known, first appeared in publication in 1980 in *The Elements of Nursing*. However, ideas and analyses are in gestation long before they ever appear in writing. That 1980 publication resulted from the establishment of 'the trio' in 1976 though, by virtue of being a coming together of like minds, much of the thinking had already been going on. Nancy Roper had by then constructed a model for nursing, and it was from this that our model was developed. The original Roper model was, in fact, an outcome of a research project undertaken between 1970 and 1974, as described in her research monograph *Clinical Experience in Nurse Education* (1976) and two other articles published that same year.

Why recount this? Well, it illustrates two points. Firstly, it contradicts the idea that models and theories are something new in Britain. Certainly the mid-1980s herald a new era, but it is not in any sense a new beginning–the Roper, Logan and Tierney model was under construction more than a decade ago.

Secondly, and more importantly, the background to this model helps to illustrate that models and theories are not developed overnight, but involve a long process–a process of construction and refinement. It is, in a sense, their very tentativeness and flexibility which permit models to help us extend our understanding of nursing. Creativity in nursing, and the pursuit of new knowledge, would simply cease were we to believe in the notion of an ultimate answer.

So the present Roper, Logan & Tierney model needs to be appreciated as a refinement and extension of the original Roper model. But the story does not stop there. The process of refinement has gone on. Even before *The Elements of Nursing* was published, work was under way on a second book, *Learning to Use the Process of Nursing* (1981). In this, what was being developed was the relationship between the model and the process of nursing–the aim being to illustrate how the model for nursing could be used as a conceptual framework, and applied in practice.

This exercise led on to the next–an attempt, albeit in a small way, to try out use of the model as a conceptual framework in nursing practice. This project involved using the model in a variety of practice settings (in hospital and community) and the nine nursing studies were carried out and written up by practising nurses, as described in the publication *Using a Model for Nursing* (1983).

Although it was only a small-scale project, and certainly not a systematic evaluation of the applicability of the model, it did provide (along with feedback from other nurses) a source of new ideas about the model and its use. Thus, the 'old' model no longer sufficed and the refined version which was developed – what is really a 'third generation' model – is presented in the second edition of *The Elements of Nursing* (1985). This version of the Roper, Logan & Tierney model will now be described, although only in outline.

Revision has been concerned with detail rather than essential characteristics of the model. A constant feature, not always recognised, is that the model for nursing is based on a model for living. Arguments supporting the rationale for linking 'nursing' and 'living' are even stronger now than before. Nurses, along with others involved in health care, are increasingly aware that people's health and the illnesses from which they suffer are inextricably linked with their lifestyle. The movement towards 'individualised nursing' demands due account to be taken of individuality in living and, recognising that most people require nursing only episodically during their lifetime, nursing should aim for minimal disruption of a person's established lifestyle.

The focus of the models is on the twelve activities of living (ALs) and, on this basis, *nursing is viewed as helping people to prevent, alleviate, solve or cope with problems related to their activities of living*. Appreciating that 'problems' may be 'potential' as well as 'actual' extends use of the model into areas of nursing activity which focus on prevention and health promotion, irrespective of whether the setting is hospital or community.

A model tends to be portrayed in diagrammatic form and a visual representation is useful because it not only highlights the main components, but also allows the relationships between and among its components to be shown. The diagrammatic representation of the Roper, Logan and Tierney model for nursing is shown in Figure 4.1.

There are five components, the first four being exactly the same in the two models (living and nursing); the unique mix of the four in the model of living contributes to 'individuality in living' and in the model of nursing to 'individualising nursing' (Table 4.1).

The model for nursing is mainly concerned with the nurse initiated part of nursing, and the visual representation in Figure 4.1 does not take account of the fact that there is a legitimate part of nursing which is derived from medical and

Table 4.1   Components of the revised model of living/model for nursing

Model of Living	Model for Nursing
* 12 activities of living	* 12 activities of living
* lifespan	* lifespan
* dependence/independence continuum	* dependence/independence continuum
* factors influencing the ALs	* factors influencing the ALs
* individuality in living	* individualising nursing

other prescription. However the nursing plan, designed for use with the model, does have a place for documentation of this delegated part of nursing; mention is made of this later.

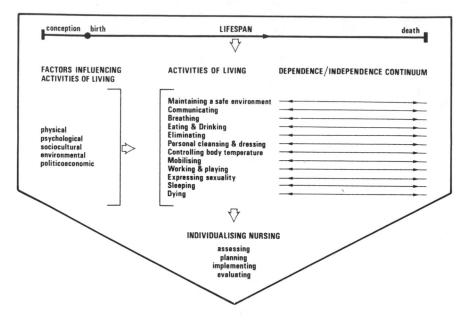

Figure 4.1   The revised (1985) Roper, Logan & Tierney model for nursing (reproduced by permission of Churchill Livingstone)

Activities of living

As said earlier, and evident in the diagrammatic representation, the activities of living (ALs) provide a focus for the models. There is, of course, nothing highly original about using the concept of 'activities of living' within a nursing model. Henderson's definition of nursing is well known and, in her exposition on the nature of nursing, she talks about basic human needs and suggests 14 'activities', although she does not use the term 'activities of living'. The set of twelve ALs in the Roper, Logan and Tierney model is, however, unique to this model.

Choosing to focus on the activities of living rather than on, for example, the concept of 'human needs' was deliberate although that too has been widely used in nursing–the advantage being that 'activities' can be described and, in some instances, measured. Calling them ALs rather than ADLs (activities of daily living) was also deliberate, as were the names decided for each of the twelve ALs. Reasons for these choices are given in *The Elements of Nursing* (1980, 1985).

The complexity of each of the ALs has to be appreciated and, as well as being complex in their own right, the 12 are closely related. For example, the AL of eating and drinking has obvious associations with the AL of eliminating. A problem with one AL may well cause problems with one or more of the others;

for example, a problem with mobilising is likely to cause problems with eliminating, personal cleansing and dressing, and working and playing.

Another dimension of the ALs is that there are priorities among them which change according to circumstances. This notion is particularly important for nursing. For example, immediately after a myocardial infarction the AL of expressing sexuality will have a low priority; but before discharge from hospital it could be of high priority as the patient wants to know whether and when it will be safe to resume sexual relations. On the other hand, for a woman scheduled for mastectomy many aspects of the same AL will be important even on admission, as well as throughout the pre- and postoperative periods, and also in the long term. What is important is for nurses to be aware that different circumstances create different priorities and, therefore, to apply common sense and professional judgement in making decisions about the relevance and relative priorities of the ALs.

The actual problems which patients may experience with the ALs are many and varied and result from a variety of causes and circumstances. Some problems result from the change of environment and routine which is an inevitable consequence of admission to hospital; others occur when illness or disability causes a change in the usual habit or mode of carrying out an AL; others are a consequence of change in the dependence/independence status; and yet another category of problems is discomforts associated with a particular AL. These groups of patients' problems and the related nursing activities are identified and discussed in the second part of each of the 12 AL chapters which make up Section 3 of *The Elements of Nursing* (1980; 1985). In the second edition, the first part of each chapter still contains an analysis of the AL in the context of healthy living but a significant addition is the discussion of the component of the model referred to as 'factors influencing activities of living' (Figure 4.1). This additional material is one of the tangible outcomes of the process of refinement of the 1980 version of the model for nursing.

Lifespan

It is easy to appreciate why lifespan is included as a second component of the model, because each person's life has a temporal dimension. 'Living' is concerned with the whole of a person's life and each person has a lifespan, however long or short. It begins at conception: birth is the event which heralds 'living' separately from the mother, and death is the event which ends the lifespan.

During life there are various stages—described, for example, as prenatal, infancy, childhood, adolescence, adulthood and old age. Each of these stages is characterised by physical, intellectual, emotional and social developments, which influence the individual's performance of the various ALs. Taking account of the patient's age—ie their stage of the lifespan—has always been recognised as important in nursing. It influences all phases of the process of nursing (assessing, planning, implementing and evaluating) and is integral to the notion of individualised nursing.

Dependence/independence continuum

The concept of dependence/independence is widely used in nursing and, as a component of this model for nursing, it relates directly to the twelve ALs. The concepts of 'dependence' and 'independence' are only meaningful as relative to one another, hence the reason for presenting these ideas by means of a continuum along which there can be movement in either direction, according to circumstance. A concept of dependence/independence applied in general to a person is too global to be meaningful, but attaching it to each AL helps to give it meaning.

Comparing the dependence/independence status of people at different stages of the lifespan illustrates the close links between these two components of the models. However, they are both necessary components because not all people are born with the potential to become independent in all 12 ALs as they progress along the lifespan. Those who are severely mentally and/or physically handicapped are in this category. Where nurses are involved in their care, at home or in an institution, the goal should be acquisition of optimal independence for each AL by carrying out an individualised programme. Other people, having gained independence in the ALs, may be deprived of it by such circumstances as accident or disease regardless of their stage on the lifespan. In these circumstances the goal is to regain as much independence as possible for the affected ALs.

Biotechnology has designed and marketed many gadgets and appliances to help those who have a congenital or acquired handicap to achieve, maintain or regain independence in particular activities. This means that nurses must accept the concept of 'aided independence' as a useful dimension of dependence/independence. It is therefore essential that the nursing documents contain adequate detail about a person's dependence/independence status for each AL, noting exactly what can and cannot be done independently, and any previous coping mechanisms—items which appear on the patient assessment form for use with the model (see later).

Developing professional judgement in relation to patients' abilities and never depriving a patient of independence in those ALs of which he or she is capable is an important skill in nursing. There is a fine dividing line between this and misjudgement in demanding independence when a person is incapable of achieving it. It is equally a skill in nursing to know when a patient is in a state of dependence; for example circumstances such as unconsciousness or severe illness when patients are totally dependent on nurses. There are other circumstances when the patient may desire to be independent but it is not in his or her best interests; such patients may need to be helped to accept that their dependence is necessary, perhaps transiently, perhaps permanently.

It cannot be stressed too strongly that a very important aspect of nursing is assessing a person's level of independence in each of the ALs and judging in which direction, and by what amount, he or she should be assisted to move along the dependence/independence continuum; what nursing help is needed to achieve the set goals; and how progress in relation to these goals will be measured and evaluated.

Factors influencing the ALs

So far three components of the model have been described; the activities of living, the lifespan and the dependence/independence continuum. Although everyone carries out activities of living at every stage of the lifespan and whatever the degree of independence, each person does so differently. To a large extent these differences arise because a variety of factors influence the way a person carries out ALs, and these 'factors' form the fourth component of the model.

It would be possible to devise a long list of different factors, such as physical; intellectual and emotional; social, religious, cultural, spiritual and ethical; environmental; political, economic and legal. Some nurses talk about 'physical, psychosocial and spiritual' dimensions. For the purposes of our model however, factors influencing the ALs are grouped into five categories:

* physical
* psychological
* sociocultural
* environmental
* politicoeconomic

Deliberately, these 'factors' are focussed on each of the 12 activities of living, as portrayed by the arrows in Figure 4.1. It would be possible to focus them on the individual as a total entity, discussing in general terms the effects of the five groups of factors on lifestyle, but this is too global. Discussing them rather as they influence each of the 12 activities of living highlights the individuality in living. Chapters 3, 4 and 5 in *The Elements of Nursing* contain information pertinent to this component of the model, and in chapters 7 to 18 each factor is discussed in relation to each AL.

Individualising nursing

This fifth component of the model for nursing derives from the 'individuality in living' component of the model of living, which itself is a product of the other four components within that model. A person's individuality can manifest itself in many different ways, as is evident from considering:

* how a person carries out the AL;
* how often the person carries out the AL;
* where the person carries out the AL;
* why the person carries out the AL in a particular way;
* what the person knows about the AL;
* what the person believes about the AL; and
* the attitude the person has to the AL.

Knowledge of a person's individuality in living is an essential prerequisite to individualising nursing. Individualised nursing can be accomplished by use of the systematic approach to patient care, what is known as 'the process of nursing'. This comprises four phases—assessing, planning, implementing and evaluating. This process is more usually referred to as the 'nursing process' but the process is not unique to nursing; it is used by many disciplines. However it is neither a 'model' nor a 'philosophy' as is sometimes written, but simply a method, and it needs to be used with an explicit nursing model. This is the rationale for incorporating the process of nursing into our model for nursing. It is the model, the conceptual framework, which provides guidelines for using the process of nursing.

The tangible evidence of whether nurses are using a model as a framework for the process of nursing–and which particular model they are using–is to be found in their documentation of a patient's nursing. To assist nurses in using the Roper, Logan & Tierney model in practice, a specially designed system of documentation has been developed. This, as illustrated in Figure 4.2, comprises:

* *A patient assessment form* on which biographical and health data and information from assessment of the twelve ALs is documented, along with related problems (actual and potential).
* *A nursing plan* –the first section for a statement of nurse-initiated interventions related to the patient's problems (actual/potential) with ALs and, the second for nursing interventions derived from medical/other prescription. In both cases there is space for documentation concerning 'goals' and 'evaluation'.

It is recommended that a separate document–sometimes referred to as 'progress notes' or 'daily notes' (we prefer the term 'patient's nursing notes')–is used over and above this specially-designed system to record additional information and actual implementation of planned interventions. This is not the place to offer detailed comment on the content and use of the proforma developed; guidelines and discussion are contained in *The Elements of Nursing* (1985).

There is nothing sacred about this particular proforma, however; it is only a guide. Nurses can devise their own documentation to suit their own practice circumstances, although obviously there is no merit in nurses in every different setting starting from scratch to devise their own documents.

Indeed, the same point could be made about the model as a whole and not just the documents. This model for nursing, as with any model, is intended as a *guide* and the hope is that nurses will use it to suit their own particular circumstances or as a starting point to further their own thinking about nursing. There is no merit, though, in each nurse developing her own model from scratch and, just as this model has grown from ideas and constructs developed by others, the intention is that it too will be modified, added to or changed, as knowledge about the discipline grows or circumstances alter. As Meleis so aptly comments; 'Looking at our theoretical present we see shadows of our past and visions of our future... the synthesis of insights of the past and visions of the future is what enhances creativity in nursing'.

There is, in the Roper, Logan & Tierney model, a combination of past and future; an amalgam of 'old' and 'new'. A model for nursing which is based on a model of living may seem to be a rather broad and somewhat simple view of nursing. In fact, this is deliberate on both counts. While acknowledging the importance and necessity of specialisation within nursing, we believe that, underlying this, there is–and should be–a consensus among nurses as to the beliefs, goals and

Figure 4.2 Patient assessment form and nursing plan (reproduced by permission of Churchill Livingstone)

Patient Assessment Form: Biographical and health data

Date of admission   Date of assessment   Nurse's signature

Surname   Forenames

Male ☐ Age ☐   Prefers to be addressed as
Female ☐ Date of birth _____
          Single/Married/Widowed/Other

Address of usual residence

Type of accommodation
(incl. mode of entry
if relevant)

Family/Others at this residence

Next of kin Name   Address

             Relationship   Tel no.

Significant others
(incl. relatives/dependants
visitors/helpers
neighbours)

Support services

Occupation

Religious beliefs and relevant practices

Recent significant life crises

Patient's perception of current health status

Family's perception of patient's health status

Reason for admission/referral

Medical information (e.g. diagnosis, past history, allergies)

GP Address Tel no.   Consultant Address Tel no.

Plans for discharge

Figure 4.2 (cont)   Patient assessment form and nursing plan (reproduced by permission of Churchill Livingstone)

Patient Assessment Form: Assessment of ALs

Date

Usual routines:
what can/cannot be done independently

Activity of living AL	previous coping mechanisms	Patient's problems: actual/potential (p)

Remainder of the
12 ALs

Maintaining a safe
  environment
Communicating
Breathing
Eating and Drinking
Eliminating
Personal cleansing
  and dressing
Controlling body
  temperature
Mobiliising
Working and playing
Expressing sexuality
Sleeping
Dying

Figure 4.2 (cont)   Patient assessment form and nursing plan (reproduced by permission of Churchill Livingstone)

Nursing Plan: Related to ALs

Goals	Nursing interventions related to ALs	Evaluation

Figure 4.2 (cont)   Patient assessment form and nursing plan (reproduced by permission of Churchill Livingstone)

Nursing Plan: Derived from medical/other prescription

Nursing interventions
derived from medical/other prescription   Goals   Evaluation

Other Notes

practices which are common to nursing, whatever the particular setting or circumstances, disease condition or patient/client group involved. Certainly for nurse learners we consider it essential that they are helped to see some connecting thread or theme to provide continuity and cohesiveness in the practice they observe and carry out in various settings, and in the various components of their theoretical instruction. Our model for nursing is, we believe, sufficiently broad and flexible to be used as a framework for the process of nursing in any area of professional practice, and as a means of appreciating the underlying unity of the various branches of the profession.

And, certainly, the model has the appearance of being simple—as simple as the model of living on which it is based. This is not to suggest that either 'living' or 'nursing' are simple processes, because of course they are not. However, we believe that to be useful a model should not be excessively complicated and, in the case of nursing, it should be directly relevant and applicable to practice. There is no necessity for a model to exhaust every aspect of the subject, and indeed, if its presentation is excessively complicated by detail, its application to practice is unlikely to be readily apparent, however interesting and academically respectable it may be. This model is not intended primarily as a theoretical construction; it is offered as a conceptual framework to assist learners to develop a way of thinking about nursing in general terms; and, in terms of its application, to be used in practice as a means of developing individualised nursing.

Menawhile, refinement of the model goes on. Even before the revised model in the new edition of *The Elements of Nursing* had reached the printer, new ideas and thoughts had surfaced. The process of constructing and refining a model is as much an outward-looking process as it is inward-looking. Much will be gained by the current climate of open debate and critical analysis of nursing models—nurses talking with model-builders and, yes, model-builders talking with each other. If there is debate and constructive criticism, based on knowledge and understanding of alternative models and theories, then so much the better for us all.

Acknowledgments

This chapter is based on the talk given by Nancy Roper and Winifred Logan at the *Senior Nurse*/Royal College of Nursing models for nursing conference held at the University of Manchester, April 1985. A revised version of the talk was published in *Senior Nurse* (3(2), July 1985). Content and illustrations based on published texts are included here with Churchill Livingstone's permission.

References

Meleis A I (1985) *Theoretical Nursing: Development and Progress*. Philadelphia: J B Lippincott Co
Nightingale F (1859) *Notes on Nursing*. Blackie, London, 1974
Roper N (1976) *Clinical Experience in Nurse Education*. Edinburgh: Churchill Livingstone
Roper N (1976) An image of nursing for the 1970s. Occasional Paper, *Nursing Times*, 29 April; 6 May

Roper N (1976) A model for nursing and nursology. *Journal of Advanced Nursing*, **1**, 219–227

Roper N, Logan W W & Tierney A J (1980) (1st Ed) (1985) (2nd Ed) *The Elements of Nursing*. Edinburgh: Churchill Livingstone

Roper N, Logan W W & Tierney A J (1981) *Learning to Use the Process of Nursing*. Edinburgh: Churchill Livingstone

Roper N, Logan W W & Tierney A J (1983) *Using a Model for Nursing*. Edinburgh: Churchill Livingstone

Models for Nursing
Edited by B Kershaw and J Salvage
©1986 John Wiley & Sons Ltd.

5

Developing and Using
a Nursing Model

STEVE WRIGHT

The academic purist might disapprove of this account of model building in the Care of the Elderly Unit at Tameside General Hospital. The story is not one of an established model being imposed as if by some God from on high. Indeed, I have strong reservations about attempts at the blanket application of one model of nursing over a wide variety of nursing settings. Models should be varied and dynamic things which help nurses in practice to explore and define their work, and should not confine them to a set order of being. Certainly, there is a need for nurses to devise systems to think about and organise their work; the process of nursing 'is not possible without a theoretical framework' (Aggleton & Chalmers 1985).

However, difficulties will arise if a model is imposed without taking account of the setting in which it is to be used. Nursing needs to adopt an eclectic approach, drawing in many ideas from theorists and model builders to produce a creative approach that is not resisted or rejected because it is seen as irrelevant to the real world of practice nurses. Such a situation could arise if, for example, the English National Board's support for and encouragement of model development in schools of nursing is interpreted rigidly as fixing a 'one and only' model policy.

Having mentioned God and the ENB, I would liken some aspects of nursing almost to a religion. It seems that whenever two or more nurses are gathered together, before they can go about the business of nursing they first ask the question, 'What is nursing?'. In trying to find the answer, nurses may end up intellectually dizzy as they spin in ever-decreasing circles. I sometimes think of nursing models as a spiral of activity. The model sets a pattern for thinking about nursing and guiding its content and practice. In doing so, more thinking and redefining takes place, so the model must change and move on as a result—and so on *ad infinitum*.

A model must never become rigid or solid, but growing and evolving structure. Input from research, practice and education must keep it alive. The contribution from nurses in practice was significant in the building of our own model at Tameside. This model building arose as a result of nurses coming together to look again at what they do–critically, sometimes cheerfully, and sometimes uncomfortably. The establishment of a joint education/service appointment was critical in creating a teaching and practising post joining both settings. Thus the job description for the joint appointee demanded 'the implementation of a model of nursing based on an individualised approach to care' (Wilkinson 1983).

A visitor to the Care of the Elderly Unit today would meet a wide spectrum of staff of very varied qualities. Until recently, few had ever heard of Henderson, Neuman, or Roper, Logan & Tierney: mention of a nursing model might have produced puzzled looks or the suggestion that perhaps it was the stuffed dummy brought in to show off the new staff uniforms. Moreover, much of the writing on models has come from the USA and many of the theorists–such as Parse, Rogers, King and Orem–often write in a style and language incomprehensible to most nurses. This can render valuable information inaccessible to the reader (Wright 1985a).

However, this is not to say that the staff I work with are anti-intellectual or do not 'think' about nursing; rather, it is that their upbringing in nursing has been academically impoverished. Their motivation and stimulation to increase their knowledge and carry out and apply research has been minimal. They are the products of a nurse education system whose failings are well documented in a multitude of reports and research (see, for example, Royal College of Nursing 1985). No model will work unless nurses are taught to be creative problem-solvers by creative teachers, practitioners and managers.

Most nurses live in communities like Tameside, where local staff of varied academic, practical and intellectual abilities nurse local people. Thus I would like to emphasise two major points:

1   Models must be built, described and used in language that is accessible to all levels of nursing staff.
2   A nursing model which focuses solely on the patient, and neglects or underestimates the nurses themselves and the social backcloth of the hospital and community, is of little value.

Furthermore, I would suggest that unless those who know about models work with those whom they would have apply them, the model can become just another piece of nursing jargon–another idea dreamed up by 'them' in cosy academic circles, with no relevance or practical application to the work setting. Then the cry will go up, 'We're not using the nursing model today because we haven't enough staff', or else the model is seen as yet another ritual like the 'back round' or 'enema days'.

Elsewhere in this volume McFarlane notes how each nurse carries with her a 'private image of nursing'. One of the steps to creating a working model of nursing is that those private worlds must be brought closer together, to work in common and as a whole. A well-established, planned strategy of changes was employed by our joint appointees so that the nurses were brought together to build their model (Lewin 1958; Ottoway 1976). The chief aim was to avoid the impression of a model being imposed from above, and the joint appointees had to take much more of a back-seat role—dropping hints or a suggestion here, mentioning a reference or a piece of research there; acting as supporters, facilitators or guides rather than dictators. There was also caution in the early stages in the choice of words used—'process', 'individualised', 'model' were out, words like 'helping with problems', 'personal' and 'ways of organising and thinking about our nursing' were in. Now words like model are adopted into our language, and I have watched with fascination as so many nurses have changed over the years in attitude and practice. Yet I suspect that most would think they themselves had changed little.

The trajectory from a medical, institutionalised, workhouse model of care to a personalised and humane one can be a long and difficult one. The option is to create a system or be dominated by another one, although to attempt change alone is dangerous. The wards and nursing communities of the UK are littered with the shattered remains of nurses who have tried to change the system alone and have been crushed. Change must be planned and organised and the change agents, be they joint appointees, charge nurses or nursing process co-ordinators, must be supported, particularly by managers and educators, if they are to succeed at the coalface. Adopting a nursing model may imply and require wholesale changes in practice; these must be pursued rationally if the cost to nurses, not least the change agents, is not to be too high (Wright 1985b).

At Tameside, the initial steps involved meetings—lots of them, talking about nursing and asking questions. The first was inevitably 'What do we believe nursing to be?'. It took four or five months alone to pull out a ward philosophy. Linchpin expressions were 'the patient's right to choose'; a view of the old person 'as a complex whole person with a right to knowledge of his or her care'; and to have nurses 'who aim to fit the setting to him or her rather than the other way round'. *The first element of the model was therefore to establish our philosophy of what nurses, nursing, and patients were.*

The deinstitutionalising effect of this questioning of the established order produced immediate, sometimes spectacular, sometimes disturbing results. As a simple example, one day a wholesale row broke out between two nursing auxiliaries. One was giving out the tea as usual (tea, sugar, milk—all in one pot). The other protested, 'But we agreed the patients have a right to choice'.

Another incident also related to the patients' right to choose. A student nurse approached me one day, looking rather anxious. She was having some difficulty adapting to a patient allocation system and felt more secure being given a list of jobs to do. The problem resolved around bathing—'I've been here two weeks and haven't bathed anybody yet'. To keep her happy, I suggested she went round and offered every patient a bath. They all refused, including one man whom the nurse felt had a very poor standard of hygiene. She tried to persuade him more firmly but was told to go away in no uncertain terms. How often, I wondered, would such a patient have been dumped in the bath whether he wanted it or not in the traditional, institutionalised, 'geriatric' setting (Wells 1980)?

Another example concerned the discussions which took place about cot sides; the staff removed them themselves when given the research/evidence for their removal, rather than being told to do so. *The second element of the model was therefore to define and provide the knowledge and skills which nurses need to nurse*, affecting both the curriculum for the statutory learners, and creating links with the continuing education department to develop relevant in-service training programmes.

Somewhere along the line words like 'process' crept in when we talked about how to put our beliefs into practice. The nurses themselves organised an 'activities of healthy living' framework for assessing and planning care. Drawing on the work of Henderson (1966) and Roper, Logan and Tierney (1980) as well as our own ideas about how we 'help' patients, *the third element of the model, the problem solving framework*, was created. The thorny problem of the documentation of the nursing process was secondary – it was developed after the pattern of care on the ward had been changed.

The spinoffs from the construction of the model encompassed the way the nursing was managed and organised, developing a patient allocation system as opposed to task allocation to make care more personal; and the way the educational curriculum was organised; the kind of research being pursued, and not least continuing developments in the practice of nursing.

The Model into education and practice

Part of the function of the joint appointees was to meet the educational needs of nursing students. If theory and practice are to be united, what students are taught about caring for the elderly must be matched by what they experience. The clinical setting must therefore not only be patient-centred but learner-centred. The development of a 'learning climate' in the ward or the classroom is essential to promote the unification of clinical and educational experience (Orton 1981).

The philosophical basis of the model provided the foundation of the students' curriculum. The following extracts from their educational aims map out the overall approach at the outset and show how the philosophy of the ward (and nursing) matched the learning approach:

> – 'The philosophy of the approach is to encourage nurses not to consider ill health as synonymous with old age, and to view ageing as a complex process of interacting physiological, psychological and sociological factors. Ageing is seen as a normal activity in the continuum of human life, in which nursing has an important helping role towards maintaining dignity, identity and independence.'
> – 'The problems perceived, both for the individual and society, will not be considered as obstructive to the sense of achievement, development and happiness which can be attained throughout the ageing years.'
> – 'The nurse will be offered an approach to care which will use the nursing model of the activities of living as a problem-solving framework, for developing the unique function of the nurse in the helping relationship with the elderly patient.'
> – 'A further purpose of the course will be to stimulate nurses to discuss and question critically their own attitudes and roles in the care of the elderly.'

−'A learning environment will be provided where learners are supported and encouraged to be actively involved both in their own learning and management of care.'

It is beyond the scope of this paper to include a full account of the educational aims and objectives, but it may be seen from these extracts, and those from the ward philosophy, that there was a sense of unity about clinical and educational aims. More precise objectives could then be developed from the activities of living framework.

Seeing ourselves as partners in care with the patient, as a specific example, some of the following objectives could be found on the subject of communications:

−'Demonstrate a role as an educator in an individual or group situation both with colleagues and with patients on the management of problems at home and on resources available in the community.'
−'Help patients to understand their care by explaining nursing care in appropriate language.'
−'Involve patients in decisions on their nursing care plans.'
−'Talk and listen to patients and relatives to help in the management of care both in hospital and at home.'

Objectives such as this must be transferred to practice. The learners, for example, help in drawing up care plans, in giving reports and in making decisions about care with patients and doctors, and they carry out the care with their allocated groups of patients. These principles can be applied to all grades of nursing staff, and care plans can be drawn up which prescribe and record the real care given to real patients. The following examples illustrate these points by showing how the model sets the guidelines which are then transferred through education into practice (Figure 5.1).

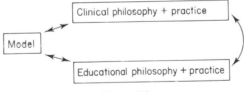

Figure 5.1

Care study 1: Jim

Jim was a fit and healthy 68-year-old who had had a 'heart attack'. There was a good chance that he could recover fully and return home. A student nurse identified some of his problems and described how she would meet his needs. (Note how the partnership, teaching and communicating concepts in the model are applied in the plan of care):

The patient's problem: Jim has had a heart attack and may get chest pains. He has never had this kind of difficulty at home before.

The nurse's aim: To minimise possible attacks of chest pain and help manage possible angina attacks at home.

Nursing care:

1   Reduce the demands of the heart through bed rest.

2   Minimise Jim's anxiety by explaining the condition, and explain all the procedures performed.

3   Observe four hourly temperatures, pulse, respiration and blood pressure to detect any deterioration.

4   Report any changes in the observations to the doctor.

5   Ask Jim to tell the nursing staff if he gets any pains.

6   Give analgesia promptly as prescribed, monitor effects with him and review with medical staff if it is ineffective.

7   Give him the *Heart Attack* booklet–giving him time to read it and then using it to teach self-management; check his understanding through questioning.

8   Spend some time sitting and talking with him–listen to what he has to say and help solve his problems through an accurate and honest account of his condition, prognosis and management.

Other aspects of Jim's care plan included the management of his gradual return to independent mobility, helping with personal hygiene while his activity was restricted and preventing bed rest complications.

The joint appointee's role, as teacher and clinician, was to help learners and others develop such plans by applying the nursing model in both its clinical and educational aspects. The fluid nature of the model also needs to be emphasised. We avoid trying to suggest that care must be written in neatly defined boxes. (The above care plan, for example, might be thought of as two problems under 'learning' and 'freedom from pain'). However, the model needs to be adaptable to help nurses think their way through care; in this instance the learner and teacher saw pain management by nurse and patient (as learning self-care) as closely and inextricably linked. Models, and the way of putting the model into action (nursing process) must not fall into the trap of becoming rigid dogma.

Care study 2: John

Following a severe stroke, John had great difficulty making his needs known. He was unable to speak, but could nod or wink to show that he understood when spoken to. The nurse planned the care with him and his relatives; some of the major points are identified as follows:

The patient's problem: John is unable to speak but appears to understand when spoken to, and is restricted in making his needs known.

The nurse's aim: To maintain effective two-way communication–to help John make his needs known and to help restore normal speech as far as possible.

Nursing care:

1   Keep the nurse call button within reach and make sure he knows where it is.

2   Explain all nursing action/care fully.

3   Provide a sign card and help John to point to things he wants.

4   Liaise with the speech therapist to assist with speech training, and follow the guidelines set.

5   Watch out for signs for things he wants, and attempt interpretation.

6   Give John time to talk–give lots of praise when he tries to speak and forms words himself.

7   Provide *Stroke Information* leaflets to John, his wife and his daughter. Give them time to read it, discuss the content and answer any questions, and encourage and teach them to participate in his care.

8   Ask the relatives to maintain visits and discuss events from home, and talk to the nurses so they know what subjects interest him.

9   Offer to help John to the day room to mix with other patients if he wishes; make sure nearby patients are aware of his difficulties and suggest simple ways they can help him.

These two care studies suggest that it is possible to build and apply a nursing model in all fields of nursing activities, to produce environments which are both patient-centred and learner-centred. The 'learner' is not just the student or pupil nurse, either; the model embodies the idea that we are all learning–patients, relatives, staff trained and untrained, regardless of setting.

I have suggested it can be difficult to change institutionalised care, and change is often measured in small steps. It may be bought at great personal expense. To those who urge the application of innovative models, I suggest caution–be supportive to those you would have change, and to those who would do the changing. When a nursing model is applied it may be in direct contravention of established laws, systems and the social order. Be mindful of what may be inflicted on the change agents when the conflicts arise over different perspectives of what nursing is between nurses, patients, relatives and other disciplines–not least the doctors, who can find a questioning, advocating nurse a disturbing prospect (Mitchell 1984).

Three support mechanisms are needed: giving help, not authoritarianism; allowing creativity and not rigid conformity to one view of nursing; and providing a credible example–being a personalising nurse and manager in practice.

Can a model be applied to break the institutional mould? Yes–but the model must reach the nurses at grass roots. We have tried in one way at Tameside, and there are others. There are many grand ideas about models, but what is needed are ways to put them into practice. When those who promote models speak up, the question must be asked–to whom do you speak? Do they listen? How can we ensure that in creating and using a model, an old woman, on a workhouse ward, in pain and grief, can be helped by nurses to the point where she can say 'yes, the nurse cares'? The ultimate test of the model is not the nurse's view, but the patient's.

References

Aggleton P & Chalmers H (1985) Paper delivered to Royal College of Nursing conference on models, reported in Caution on nursing theory bandwagon. *Nursing Times*, **81**(40), 8

Henderson V (1966) *The Nature of Nursing*. New York: MacMillan

King I M (1971) *Toward a Theory of Nursing*. New York: John Wiley & Sons

Lewin K (1958) The group decision and social change. In Maccoby E (ed) *Readings in Social Psychology*. New York: Holt, Rinehart & Winston

Mitchell J R A (1984) Is Nursing Any Business of Doctors? A Simple Guide to the Nursing Process. *British Medical Journal*, **288**, 216–219

Neuman B (1980) The Betty Neuman health-care systems model: a total person approach to viewing patient problems. In Riehl J & Roy C (eds) *Conceptual Models for Nursing Practice*. New York: Appleton-Century-Crofts

Orem D E (1980) *Nursing–Concepts of Practice*. New York: McGraw-Hill

Orton H (1981) *The Ward Learning Climate*. London: Royal College of Nursing

Ottoway R M (1976) A change strategy to implement new norms, new style and new environment in the work organisation. *Personal Review*, **5**(1), 1 & 3

Parse R R (1981) *Man–Living–Health–A Theory of Nursing*. New York: John Wiley & Sons

Rogers M E (1970) *The Theoretical Basis of Nursing*. Philadelphia: F A Davis

Roper N, Logan W & Tierney A (1980) *The Elements of Nursing*. Edinburgh: Churchill Livingstone

Royal College of Nursing Commission on Nursing Education (1985) *The Education of Nurses–A New Dispensation*. London: RCN

Wells T (1980) *Problems in Geriatric Nursing*. Edinburgh: Churchill Livingstone

Wilkinson K (1983) A blueprint for a joint appointment. *Nursing Times*, 19 October

Wright S G (1985a) It's all right in theory... *Nursing Times*, **81**(34), 19–20

Wright S G (1985b) Change in nursing: the application of change theory to practice. *Nursing Practice*, **1**(2)

Wright S G (1985c) A Rich Experience. *Nursing Times*, **81**(36), 38–39

Models for Nursing
Edited by B Kershaw and J Salvage
© 1986 John Wiley & Sons Ltd.

6

Nursing Models and Multidisciplinary Teamwork

ALAN PEARSON

Those who advocate the use of a conceptual model for nursing in practice list a number of advantages in doing so. One is that a clear description of what nurses see as the province of nursing defines the role of the nurse in relation to the patient and the other disciplines which make up the multidisciplinary team (Pearson & Vaughan 1986). Here I would like to relate model-based practice to the nurse in the multidisciplinary clinical team.

Multidisciplinary teamwork is becoming widely accepted as a desirable aim in caring for the elderly, as well as in psychiatry, paediatrics and primary health care. Batchelor (1980) comments that, outside psychiatry, 'it would be rare ... for any doctor who was not a geriatrician to consider himself a member of a multidisciplinary team in any formal sense', although it could be said from experience that true multidisciplinary teamwork is still not the norm even in elderly care settings. The combination of active therapies, nurturing, caring and investigative procedures which are needed to meet the needs of the elderly person points to the absurdity of assuming that one particular discipline should be the unequivocal leader of others. A team of people with a variety of backgrounds and skills is increasingly being seen as the core of good practice. All who have an input to care need to be drawn into a co-operative effort to help the patient, and all have an important therapeutic role.

Multidisciplinary teamwork in health care

The sick, disabled, or vulnerable person who becomes a receiver of any form of health care today inevitably faces a huge variety of health care workers, who all have a part to play in helping them to achieve as healthy a state as possible. The effective care of all patients or clients; their satisfaction with care; and their understanding of it; depends on a large group of people with very different views

47

and expertise. If each one works independently doing her bit and paying little attention to the other members of the team, care will be disjointed and virtually chaotic.

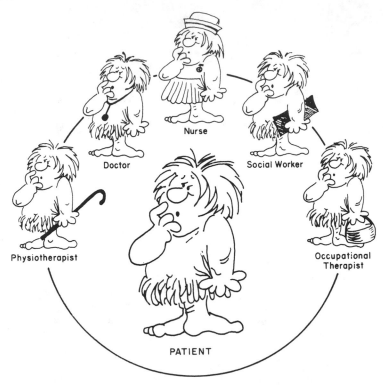

Figure 6.1   The multidisciplinary clinical team

On the whole health workers do not work in total isolation, but there is increasing evidence that conflict frequently arises between members of multidisciplinary teams, and that it may be difficult to deliver care because of the number of types of health worker and the confusion concerning the role of the nurse (Benne and Bevis 1959). Take, for example, the routine admission of an elderly, articulate and normally independent woman to an elderly care ward for rehabilitation following a stroke. She arrives on the ward and is met by the *ward clerk*, who asks a good deal of questions and records the answers in writing, and then asks her to wait until she seeks a nurse. A young man in a white coat arrives, says he is a *nurse*, and shows her to her bed. After getting undressed, she meets, over the course of two days, a lot of other nurses, two *sisters*, four *doctors*, a *phlebotomist*, a *dietician*, a *physiotherapist*, an *ECG technician*, three *domestics*, two *porters*, a *radiographer* and an *occupational therapist*. Apart from the whole team of nurses who have come and gone over these 48 hours, this potentially vulnerable person has met 19 different people. If she has more specific problems, she may well meet even more, such as a social worker or stoma therapist–and the list could go on. Worse still, all could work in conflicting ways. No matter how skilled or empathetic each member of a team is, the sort of care needed by this imaginary woman, or any receiver of health care, cannot be given until the team as a whole knows what each member is contributing and what information is being given.

Most patients receive health care from more than one type of worker. The patient attending his GP's surgery with a common cold may only need to see the doctor, while the woman at home with a hemiplegia may need the help of a community nurse, social worker, physiotherapist and occupational therapist. The composition of the team therefore varies according to the needs of the patient, but consists of those workers who contribute to the overall health care of the individual. The notion of this team has been around for some years, particularly in primary health care, and is based on the broader concept of team effort–team being defined as a group of people who work together towards a common goal.

Each member of a team must have a specific contribution to make to the overall achievement of the objective, although strict boundaries between what each can or cannot do is not necessarily important; the patient/client is always the most important member of the team. To function effectively, each member including the patient should know what the others are contributing towards the objective, and must value their contributions. Failure leads to disjointed action, non-achievement of the agreed goal, and conflict.

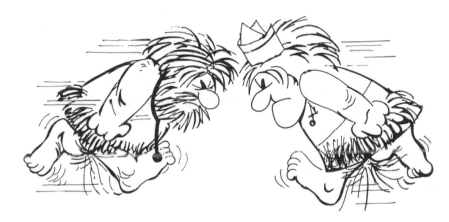

Figure 6.2   When team members don't know or understand the contributions of others

The patient who has just suffered a stroke with a resulting hemiplegia, for example, may need a team of workers whose objective is to enable him to be relatively independent in his daily living and to have a blood pressure within defined normal limits. The patient contributes himself and his knowledge of his capabilities and desires. The doctor contributes expertise in diagnosing the cause of the paralysis, treating it and preventing a recurrence. The nurse contributes expertise in carrying out daily activities for the patient until he is able to do so himself, enabling him to make sense of what has happened to him and monitoring progress. The physiotherapist contributes expertise in restoring the actions of some of the affected muscles, motivating him to reclaim lost mobility and activity, and providing suitable aids to mobility. The occupational therapist contributes expertise in teaching new ways of achieving activities of daily living, assessing for and providing suitable aids, and in advising on the design and operation of alterations in living areas to allow maximum independence. Finally, the social worker contributes expertise in assessing social needs, identifying and mobilising community and governmental resources and developing relationships between the patient and meaningful others (Pearson 1985). Thus each member of the team has a special contribution towards the goal of the team, although they work together in such a way that their actions often overlap; for example, the occupational therapist may involve the nurse in the use of a specific aid. All operate from different but complementary models for practice.

The doctor's view that the patient may need to lie flat for 24 hours influences the actions of the others; and the nurse's view that to do so will lead rapidly to high anxiety or a breakdown of the skin will influence whether the doctor's view should be followed. Discussion within the team allows a rational and logical decision to be reached by weighing up the pros and cons identified through corporate expertise.

Most of us are already a part of a team such as this, be it in a hospital, the community, or an industrial setting, and we recognise that the principles outlined are desirable. Yet misunderstanding and excessive dominance by one group of professionals, and therefore a less rosy picture, are not uncommon. The secretariat of the Royal Commission on the NHS (1980) recognised a number of difficulties and obstacles to teamwork in the NHS, and held that the difficulties seen in a multidisciplinary team approach were more attributable to interprofessional jealousies than to anything more solid.

The notion of teamwork is therefore logical and attractive, but does not naturally seem to lead to the widespread adoption of the multidisciplinary team approach. The development of teams of mammoth proportions means, however, that greater clarity about each other's contributions cannot reasonably be expected to occur without a belief in the principles of the team.

All teams are, of course, different, and subject to changes in membership, either because of members leaving or because of the needs of individual patients. A standard recipe to improve communications is therefore impossible, although there are a number of ideas which may lead to greater cohesion and better communication.

If nurses are to participate effectively in the multidisciplinary team, it is essential that they agree on an explicit model for practice. All members of practice disciplines hold a model in their head, and although there are variations between each person, occupational groups usually share a common understanding of their own discipline. The components of a model have been described in a number of ways. One analysis suggests that a model for practice tells the world what the practitioner believes about the nature of the client; what the goals of practice are; and what the practitioner needs to know in order to achieve these goals (Pearson & Vaughan 1984). In the health team, it is commonly assumed that the doctor believes the patient to be a physiological being susceptible to illness, disease, or disability; the goal of medical practice is to cure such disorders, or to relieve the symptoms when cure is not feasible; and the knowledge needed stems from the biological sciences. Similarly, the physiotherapist can readily identify the components of the commonly accepted model of his or her practice.

In nursing, however, its neglect of theorising and its obsession with 'doing' without thought have meant there is no commonly accepted model. Furthermore, the huge differences in the settings and client groups associated with nursing make it impossible ever to arrive at such an all-embracing model. However, an abundance of models specific to nursing is now available to suit many of the fields in which nurses practice. It is possible for a team of nurses on a ward or in the community to agree on a model which reflects to them the reality of their practice. Ruddock (1972) says that 'models are aids to thinking, and in respect of some problems may be a necessary condition for thought'. The all too common problem of nurses' inability to become an equal member of the team may partly be overcome through the nurses involved agreeing on an appropriate practice model, and then making this explicit to the other disciplines. In any team the members who are unable to establish a role which contributes to the team's effort in the same way as other members will not be valued, and their expertise will be underused.

Using a model in multidisciplinary practice

I work in a small integrated unit in a rural area. It consists of 12 inpatient beds, outpatients, a day hospital, a casualty department, a district nursing service and a health visiting service, and also serves the health authority as a research and development unit. Its major brief in this respect is to develop clinical nursing by exploring and innovating in activities of direct patient care, and by trying to develop nursing practice which also includes teaching and research and has a sound knowledge base. Until four years ago the unit was an ordinary cottage hospital with very traditional practices, not least the domination of the health care team by medical practitioners. Much has changed since, stemming directly from the initial educational programme for nursing staff which led them to learn about a variety of nursing models and finally agree on one which they felt described nursing adequately, and with which they could identify. The exercise itself was more important than the specific model chosen, which was the activities of living model described by Roper, Logan & Tierney (1980).

This model has worked well because the nurses using it chose it themselves as a basis for practice and agreed to use it as a nursing team. Its adoption, however, was not quite as easy as you might imagine. The model did demand a change in practice; for example, it required an effective assessment of the client, which included exploring thorny areas like sexuality and death. In our initial attempts to do this, conflict arose with other disciplines. Doctors didn't want nurses to ask such things of *their* patients, while occupational therapists felt that assessing activities of living was an intrusion on their role. To help resolve the conflict we held multidisciplinary workshops using role play and feedback, run by North West Spanner, the Manchester-based theatre company which had previously taught empathy skills to nurses (Swaffield 1982; Whitehouse *et al* 1984). The experience led to a really important change in attitudes to teamwork; confirmed much that has already been written about how to pursue it; and verified the overwhelming need for any team of nurses to be explicit about their beliefs about patients, their perceived goals of nursing and their skills and knowledge.

The focus of the workshops was the patient, rather than the professional status or role defensiveness of the health workers. The major learning, however, related to an understanding of the different yet complementary contributions made to overall care by the primary nurses practising in the hospital. These nurses felt secure in their roles because they worked in a nurse-orientated environment where there had been considerable development of professional status since practice had become based on an explicit model (Pearson *et al* 1985). This account of these sessions nevertheless noted continuing conflict between health visitors and other disciplines; the health visitors were unable to state clearly their beliefs and values about clients, their overall goals of practice, or the knowledge needed to achieve them. The team were eventually able to acknowledge that nursing was in reality different to their former perception of it, and that nurses' contribution to patient care was different to other disciplines. The nurses clearly, confidently and unanimously presented the Roper, Logan & Tierney model as a description of the way in which they practised.

The multidisciplinary team agreed that the model did represent nursing, and accepted that the role of the nurse was to function on this basis. The process of thinking about the nature of nursing through looking at various models, and then agreeing as a group on an overall framework, led to greater cohesion and interest among the nurses themselves; extending this exercise to the rest of the team led to greater role clarity and cohesion. There were direct benefits to patients, because effective teamwork is an essential precursor of quality performance.

In practice, total compliance with nurses' views does not and never should prevail; but their expertise and difference in focus is acknowledged. Clashes between nurses and doctors are inevitable and, indeed, more likely now that they are clear about their concerns for patients, and confident of their right to pursue them. For example, the desire to help a patient achieve independence may lead him and his nurse to pursue a plan which involves high risks, such as the removal of cot sides, which may conflict with the doctor's view of preventing possible mishaps. Conflict arose between the same two disciplines when a patient with a lifelong drinking habit was admitted for terminal care. The medical perspective focused on prolonging life, and took the line that no alcohol should be available.The nurse, concerned with preserving the patient's usual life style and helping him maintain his independence, strongly disagreed. In the past both examples might have been regarded as emotive opinions held by the nurse because of her 'nature'. Now, although the nurse's view may not be agreed with, it is more often seen as a perspective based on a rationally developed conceptual framework.

At this stage in the development of British nursing, ward or community nursing teams should be encouraged to study the various models and to agree on one suitable for practice in their area which 'grabs' the specific team. While an eclectic approach may be ideal, and while it may be better for nurses to apply appropriate models to individual patients, this is not a practical course to pursue at present. Real nurses nursing real patients are busy, tired, and therefore unable to engage in elaborate conceptual exercises throughout the working day. Indeed, a good model for practice helps us to organise knowledge and approach problems in the face of obstacles and the need to make difficult decisions.

A move towards model-based practice is the most important target for change today. It precedes all other innovations–I see little point in introducing problem-orientated records in a nursing unit without first agreeing on a model for practice. I see no point in discussing the accountability of individual nurses until the team has a shared understanding of what nursing is. I see no value in discussing the extended role of the nurse until the current role can be understood through agreeing on a model which describes nursing. All our hopes for change directed at improving the service of nurses to patients hinge on individual nursing teams actively exploring the act of nursing by considering the concept and descriptions of nursing models. All nursing teams should be encouraged and helped to identify an appropriate model, and then to share their decision with the wider multidisciplinary team.

My experience suggests that this is vital to effective teamwork aimed at high quality patient care. Although we are not quite there yet, the use of a model in our unit is increasing the other members' understanding of the nursing contribution and making them value nursing more highly. I hope this will produce good teamwork and occasional harmony between disciplines.

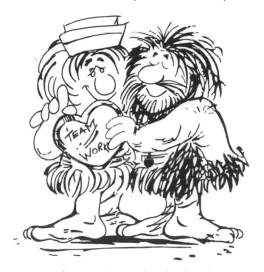

Figure 6.3   When team members understand and value the contributions of others

References

Batchelor I (1980) *The Multi-disciplinary Team–A Working Paper*. London: King's Fund

Benne K & Bevis W (1959) Role confusion and conflict in nursing: the role of the professional nurse. *American Journal of Nursing*, 59(2), 196–198

Pearson A (1985) Getting it right: interprofessional communication. *Nursing*, **2**(38), June

Pearson A, Morris P & Whitehouse C (1985) Consumer-oriented groups: a new approach to interdisciplinary teaching. *Journal of the Royal College of General Practitioners*, 35, 381–383

Pearson A & Vaughan B M (1984) In *A Systematic Approach to Nursing Care*. Milton Keynes: Open University

Pearson A & Vaughan B (1986) *Nursing Models in Practice*. London: Heinemann

Roper N, Logan W & Tierney A (1980) *The Elements of Nursing*. Edinburgh: Churchill Livingstone

Ruddock R (ed) (1972) *Six Approaches to the Person*. London: Routledge & Kegan Paul

Secretariat of the Royal Commission (1980) *Multidisciplinary Clinical Teams–History and Development*. London: King's Fund

Swaffield L (1982) Spanner in the works. *Nursing Times*, **78**, 1049–1054

Whitehouse C R, Morris P & Marks B (1984) The role of actors in teaching communication. *Medical Education*, **18**, 62–68

North West Spanner can be contacted c/o Penny Morris, 6 Lombard Grove, Fallowfield, Manchester

Models for Nursing
Edited by B Kershaw and J Salvage
© 1986 John Wiley & Sons Ltd.

7

A Stress Adaptation Model

GEORGE CASTLEDINE

'Which should come first, the nursing process or a model of nursing?' In practice, the answer to this question has proved three things: firstly, that nursing process and models of nursing are not the same thing, but are different; secondly, nursing process can be used as a vehicle to bring about the application of a model, showing their inter-relatedness; thirdly, nursing theory can be incorporated as an integral part of nursing practice as long as there is commitment, knowledge, understanding and flexibility.

I pose the above question because I was faced with this problem just over 10 years ago, when I was about to change the style of management of nursing care on a hospital ward. Over the years the same question has kept appearing in many different clinical settings, in hospital and the community. Writing from my experience of applying the nursing process and acting as a consultant in nursing, I hope this chapter will help the student (both qualified and unqualified) come to terms with some of the difficulties posed by nursing process and nursing model application.

My main objectives here are:

to outline the historical development of the move to apply nursing process and integrate it with a model of nursing,
to summarise the key factors of the Roy adaptation model, and
to discuss the ways in which the Roy adaptation model was adopted and changed to suit the various needs of nursing practice.

From nursing process to a model of nursing

Before changing any system of nursing care, be it in hospital or in the community, it is important to find out how good or bad that system is. In many ways you are simply applying the nursing process or problem-orientated approach to the nursing setting; and if you do not know what you are changing from, you will have difficulty in determining that you have achieved something new and different.

Through examining the nursing records you will identify strengths and weaknesses in the nurses' written abilities and nursing knowledge base. If a system of nursing process is already in progress there should be evidence of some kind of assessment by a nurse of the patient's nursing condition. Problems should be clearly stated and care plans should show how prescriptions of nursing care have been applied. There should be evidence that the patient is involved in making progress. Overall what should be found is a blueprint or a picture of the patient from the nursing point of view. Also, by observing and listening to report sessions about the patients the change agent will soon be able to evaluate the strengths and weaknesses of the nursing staff, their attitudes and commitment to change.

The type of patients and their medical and nursing problems must be considered. Is their contact with nurses going to be over a long or a short period of time, for instance? In many acute hospitals rapid patient turnover influences the depth of information needed, and thus the use of nursing process and a model of care. Ward layout and design may also be important factors, and assessment should be made of the nursing equipment available. In the community, the size of the nurse's caseload is important, as is the support the clients receive from family and friends. The accessibility of clinic facilities or emergency hospital beds is also relevant.

These and many other factors should be thought through carefully before any change is introduced. Unless extensive consideration is given to strategies for change, the introduction of any new method or management style will fail.

Two main problems are evident in the successful implementation of change in nursing. Firstly, adjustments necessary in moving towards a nursing process approach either are not recognised, or are resisted by a desire to maintain the *status quo*. Secondly, nurses lack the knowledge and more particularly the skills needed to use nursing process (Table 7.1).

Owing to the previous emphasis in nursing education on tasks and physical procedures, nurses in the UK are very good at psychomotor skills. It is important, however, to encourage all members of the nursing team to update and review their affective and cognitive skills.

The way that change is introduced, enforced and timed is critical to its success. It would be too dogmatic to state how the nursing process or model development should be introduced into the clinical setting. Each setting where nursing is practised is different, and like the patient each should be treated individually and respectfully.

Evaluating and preparing the clinical setting were key factors in the development of the adaptation model. The next stage was the identification of patients' problems. This was achieved by encouraging the nurses to write down on the records what they felt the patients' nursing requirements to be. The result was a list of medical factors relating and, on many occasions, including the medical diagnosis. When they were invited to compile a nursing assessment form, much of the information was again focused on the patients' possible medical diagnosis. There was also great emphasis on the need for information on such topics as

Table 7.1   Skills for Nursing Process (some factors)

Cognitive (intellectual)
>   Systematic thinking
>   Experience of life
>   Experience in nursing
>   General education
>   Post-basic and continuing education
>   Critical thinking
>   Judgement
>   Insight

Interpersonal (affective)
>   Ability to develop rapport with people
>   Ability to develop nurse/client relationships
>   Empathic listening
>   Transmission of caring and feeling
>   Mutual trust and rapport
>   Creativity (ability to test new and original approaches)
>   Adaptability (flexibility and a willingness to consider alternatives)
>   Interview skills
>   Observation skills
>   Consultation and counselling skills

Technical skills (psychomotor)
>   Ability to perform techniques, procedures and methods
>   Manipulation of special equipment and instruments
>   Ability to examine and handle patients physically and their equipment such as
>   wheel chairs and walking aids

the patients' valuables and biographical details, because of the rules and regulations of the hospital.

Wherever the nursing process is developed, there is a danger that what will emerge is a systematic routine method of collecting patient information which may well conform to legal and institutional demands, but is superficial and irrelevant to nursing care. If nurses are unsure about the type of information to collect, it is important to have guidelines or a teaching aid. At this point we explored the use of a model of nursing.

In the mid-1970s there were very few guides and little information on which model of nursing to choose. However, the first edition of Riehl and Roy's *Conceptual Models for Nursing Practice* had just been published. The choice of an adaptation model was not based on the fact that it was easy to understand, but that I strongly agreed with its underlying assumptions.

Adaptation

It has been said that adaptation is the expression of human interaction with the environment. According to Lewontin (1978), the modern view of adaptation is that 'the external world sets certain "problems" that organisms need to "solve", and that evolution by means of natural selection is the mechanism for creating these solutions'. This author is suggesting that adaptation is the process of evolutionary change by which an organism provides a better or improved solution to its problems. Becoming adapted is the end result. A key is adapted to a lock by cutting and filing, an electrical appliance is adapted to a different voltage by a transformer, and an old house is adapted for modern living. Biologists define adaptation according to a particular environment. Anthropologists add the dimension of changing the environment through cultural means in such a manner that it is better suited to human needs. The nursing view is probably well summed up by Beland (1981), who defines adaptation as 'the temporary or permanent changes in structure, function, behaviour or culture that enable an individual or group to survive in a particular environment'.

Table 7.2   Comparison of the Components of the Medical and Nursing Adaptation Models (adapted from Rambo 1984)

Components	Medical model	Stress/nursing adaptation model
Recipient	Sick person, any age	Person, any age, sick or well any-where on the health-illness conti-nuum with a coping problem
Approach	Problem-solving method (ie. scientific)	Problem-solving method (ie. nursing)
Focus of services	Cellular changes and symp-toms caused by disease and trauma	Coping problems influenced by location on the health-illness continuum
Goal	Cure	Promote adaptation in all ways possible and interdependence
Intervention		
Setting	Office, clinic, hospital or or other health care agency	Anywhere: home, community, hospital or health care agency
Procedure; process	Medical process to diagnose and prescribe treatment	Nursing process, to assess behaviours, identify problems, and intervene by manipulating stimuli
Agent for change	Physician/surgeon	Patient or client (with help from nurse) as an adaptive being
Source of energy	Physician acts upon patient, with medication and therapy given by others	Patient's coping mechanisms sup-ported by problem-solving nurse

Environment is an important factor, it would seem, in relation to adaptation. Beland sees it as a response that favours survival in a particular environment—different to tolerance in that it is a positive response. Tolerance is accomplished by a loss of function.

There are several key biological mechanisms of adaptation, such as cell division under stress, genetic mutation, and the response of the immune system. There are good examples of human adaptation in body build—for example the short, stocky Eskimos, and the long thin trunks of Africans. People who live at high altitude develop an increased chest size. Examples of temporary adaptation are tanning of the skin and increase in muscle size for certain types of sport. Exposure to sickle cell anaemia in Africa reduces the chance of malaria, and the growing number of people with essential hypertension as an adaptation to society's stressful living is a form of adaptation.

Factors which seem to influence the capacity of the individual to adapt are genetic constitution (heredity); the ability to meet physiological and psychosocial needs; anatomical integrity and a reduction in bodily defects; learning and experiencing–exposure and education are important; and age (the old have greater difficulty in adapting). There are several characteristics of adaptation, and it would seem that the whole organism or person has to be involved in order to adapt. The amount of energy of a person appears to affect their adaptation–hence the need to 'nourish' sick people. Finally, as Beland points out, 'there is a range to the capacity to adapt; when this range is exceeded, health or even life is threatened.'

The Roy adaptation model

Roy (1980) develops this theme of adaptation and applies it to nursing. Her model contains eight basic assumptions, as follows:

1   The person is a biopsychosocial being.
2   The person is in constant interaction with a changing environment.
3   The person uses innate and acquired mechanisms, which are biologic, psychologic, and social in origin.
4   Health and illness are an inevitable dimension of the person's life.
5   The person must adapt to respond positively to environmental changes.
6   The person's adaptation is a function of the stimulus he or she is exposed to and of his or her adaptation level.
7   The person's adaptation level is such that it comprises a zone indicating the range of stimulation that will lead to a positive response.
8   The person is conceptualized as having four modes of adaptation: physiologic needs, self-concept, role function, and interdependence relations.

Roy proposes two further assumptions in regard to the self-concept mode. These are that the self-concept arises out of perception and is the product of social reaction, and that self-concept has a predictable effect on behaviour.

Fitzpatrick and Whall (1983) point out that the soundness of assumptions can be assessed using the three levels of assumptions identified by Fox (1970). First level assumptions are the soundest, and have their foundations in previous research. Second level assumptions are those which stem from general theory, particularly if empirical data indicate that the theory has substance. Third level assumptions are based on the personal experience of the researcher and others.

Assumptions 1 to 7 of the model can be classified as second level assumptions. These stem from theory in physiologic psychology, psychology, sociology and nursing, and there are empirical data to indicate that this general theory base has substance. The two additional assumptions can also be classified as second level assumptions and are derived from theories of growth and development, motivation and learning.

Assumption 8 is the weakest and would be classified as third level; it is based on the experience of Roy and others. Roy (1970, 1980) analyzed 500 samples of patient behaviours collected by nursing students, and then proposed that human beings have four adaptive modes.

The central components of all nursing models appear to be the concepts of person, nursing, health and environment (Figure 7.1a). In Roy's model there are five elements, all affected by adaptation theory (Figure 7.1b), as follows:

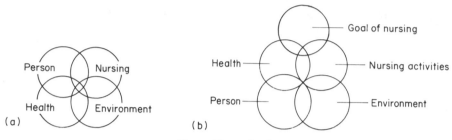

Figure 7.1a and 7.1b

1   *Person* – could be seen not only as the individual but a family, group, community or society. All are adaptive systems and all vary according to situations and circumstances.

2   *Health* – not just seen as a continuum but relating to the process of becoming an integrated 'whole', ie. a holistic approach.

3   *Environment* – people exist in an open environment and also have an internal bodily environment to cope with.

4   *Nursing activity* – nurses act by manipulating the focal, contextual and residual stimuli or main causes, so that a person can adapt positively.

5   *Goal of nursing* – the promotion of adaptive responses in relation to the four adaptive modes, the physical, self-concept, role function and interdependence.

The components of the model to which she gives most emphasis are the concepts of the person as an adaptive system, and adaptation. She views health as a continuum which varies for each person, but contains an inevitability that one day he or she will become ill. It is important that when the inevitable happens, ie. sickness, the person responds by adapting positively and returning to good health.

Beland sees the nurse's responsibilities in this adaptation approach as assessing the person's adaptive capacity, modifying the environment so that he or she is protected from excessive demands, and assisting him or her in utilising adaptive capacities for his or her own benefit. Roy would probably agree with this, and emphasises that the person has four areas or modes which are crucial in their adaptation to illness. These are basic physiological needs, self-concept, role function and interdependence. She says the nurse must assess these areas in each patient, and in doing so must try to identify positive and negative behaviours in the four modes. The positive behaviours are reinforced and the negative behaviours are hopefully changed by utilising the stages of the nursing process.

First table:

First Level Assessment			Second Level Assessment			Nursing Diagnosis	Intervention		
Assessment Factors	Behaviour		Stimuli				Goals	Approach	Evaluation
	Positive	Negative	Focal	Contextual	Residual				
Physical Needs									
Self Concept									
Role Function									
Inter Dependence									

Figure 7.2 The diagram above shows how Wagner (1976) interpreted Roy and the nursing process. The UK approach as devised by Castledine is shown in the lower diagram.

Second table:

First Level Assessment			Second Level Assessment			Problem Statement or Nursing Diagnosis*	Nursing Plans			
Assessment Factors	Behaviour		Stimuli				Goals or Outcomes	Nursing Interventions	Progress Notes	Evaluation
	Positive	Negative	Focal	Contextual	Residual					
Physical Needs										
Self Concept										
Role Function										
Inter Dependence										

* Stated, if possible, in patient terms

Figure 7.3   Nursing assessment (use of Roy's first-level assessment)

Assessment Factors	Behaviour	
	Positive	Negative
I		
PHYSICAL BASIC NEEDS		
A **Exercise and Rest**		
1. Immobility		
2. Fatigue		
B **Nutrition**		
1. Malnutrition		
2. Feeding		
3. Nausea and vomiting		
C **Elimination**		
Urinary incontinence		
Faecal incontinence		
D **Fluids and Electrolytes**		
Dehydration		
E **Oxygen and Circulation**		
Hypoxia		
Stasis		
F **Regulation**		
1. Temperature		

Figure 7.3 (cont) Nursing assessment (use of Roy's first-level assessment)

Assessment Factors	Behaviour	
	Positive	Negative
F continued		
2. Senses		
a) altered sensation		
b) sensory deprivation		
c) pain		
3. Endocrine system		
II SELF CONCEPT MODE		
a) Physical self loss		
b) Anxiety		
c) Powerlessness		
III ROLE FUNCTION		
IV INTERDEPENDENCE		

Another attractive aspect of the Roy model is its suggestion of two levels of assessment. This involves the nurse not only in identifying the positive and negative behaviours of the patient (first level), but in trying to identify in greater depth the main stimuli which were causing the positive or negative reactions (second level). Figure 7.2 shows an overview of this first and second level of assessment leading to a nursing diagnosis or statement of the patient's problems, intervention and evaluation.

In Roy's adaptation model, the physiologic mode relates to physical needs such as exercise and rest, nutrition, elimination, fluid and electrolytes, oxygen, circulation and regulation, including temperature, the senses and the endocrine system. The self-concept mode includes the composite of beliefs and feelings held about the self at a given time, formed particularly from perceptions of others' reactions, and directing personal behaviour. In the third key area, role function, a role defines the expected behaviours a person should perform to maintain a title. Finally, interdependence concerns the comfortable balance between dependence and interdependence in relationships with others.

The three main stimuli noted in the second level assessment are focal, contextual and residual. The focal stimulus is the degree of change or stimulus most immediately confronting the person and the one to which they must make an adaptive response; that is, the cause of the behaviour. Contextual stimuli are factors which may be affecting behaviour but whose effects are not validated.

Adapting the adaptation model

To adapt or modify something implies some form of change in quality, so it fits more easily that which was intended. In applying the adaptation approach to nursing and the Roy model in particular, we set out to seek the balance between fitting the model to nursing practice and fitting the nursing practice to the model. How did we use in practice the first level assessment of the Roy model? Although we recorded the first level assessment data about patients, because of limited time we did not add the information relating to the stimuli. When we had time, however, we did discuss this information.

The forms we used for developing the assessment stage of the Roy model are shown in Figure 7.3. Headings were used so that the nurse could develop her ideas without feeling too restrained by 'yes or no' answers or ticking boxes, as found on some other nursing assessment forms. The other forms included a nursing care plan containing separate columns for nursing problems, goals and objectives of care and a nursing plan, and finally an evaluation sheet. These papers were kept separate in a large file and used in conjunction with the ward Kardex system. Every new member of the nursing team underwent our own nursing process training programme, which included a general talk, discussion and a handout of the type of information we were looking for and wanted included in our process papers. We allocated nurses to individual patients and encouraged them to use the process with that person. This resulted in us having to support some nurses continually, but in the majority of cases, irrespective of stage of training, they completed this task admirably. Sometimes assessments were carried out immediately on a patient's admission to the ward, and sometimes later. Most information was gathered with direct permission from the patient, but on certain occasions—for example, if the patient was unconscious—information was sought from relatives and friends. By adopting this approach we felt we were seeking some form of uniformity in our communication purposes, and at the same time allowing maximum flexibility to encourage students and ward staff to be creative in their thinking.

A common misconception used as an excuse for not carrying out total patient care is that each ward needs a very high staffing level. We allocated one nurse to one or two patients for making an assessment and planning care, but because of staffing fluctuations we expect our staff to work with up to 15 patients on one shift. This means that several nurses will be involved in implementing and evaluating a particular patient's care plan.

It is important to have regular reporting and discussion sessions with all staff to help in evaluating and reassessing a patient's care plan. These vary according to the patients and ward staff's needs; for example, we carried out at least two main reporting sessions a day and one patient-orientated care conference a month. The former involves the nurses who have been in charge of a particular group of patients handing over the care plans to the oncoming staff. The latter involves an extended, hour-long review of one or two patients' care, pointing out such issues as medical involvement, physiotherapy, community and associated para-nursing care.

The present adaptation model has been designed for use in various fields of nursing. It has been tried out in practice, but as yet no serious evaluation of its effectiveness has been carried out. There are three main areas of patient assessment, all of which can be carried out at a first level (superficial) or second level (in depth).

The first area of assessment involves the patient's biographical and general social details (Figure 7.4). The second involves physical condition and needs, and the third relates to the psychosocial state. When assessing in the second and third areas, the nurse is encouraged to use a holistic approach and identify both positive and negative aspects. The emphasis on the stimuli which cause the positive and negative behaviours is not as detailed as that in Roy's original work. The identification of the causes of such behaviour is encouraged, and where possible developed at evaluation sessions with the patient, care conferences and report sessions.

There are two methods of carrying out a physical examination, the second area of patient assessment. The first is a head-to-toe approach similar to that suggested in Figure 7.5. The second is a major body systems approach, covering the following areas: general information, skin, eyes, ears, respiratory functions, the cardiovascular system, the gastrointestinal system, the urinary system, the nervous system and the musculoskeletal system.

The third area of patient assessment, looking at psychosocial state, deals with intrapersonal, interpersonal and interdependency assessments. The intrapersonal assessment involves self-concept, such as body image, body, self ideal and esteem; cognition, including reality orientation; affect and mood, such as anxiety, anger and depression; pain; and spiritual/belief feelings. The interpersonal assessment looks at body language; stress and stressors; coping mechanisms; role function; adaptation to the patient role; and relationships with others. The interdependence assessment identifies dependent and independent behaviours, and attention and affection seeking.

Figure 7.4 First area of patient assessment

General and Biographical Information

Surname: _____ Forenames: _____

Address: _____

Next of kin: _____ Date of birth: _____

Age: _____

Relevant Tel. Nos: _____

Close friends and family: _____

Likes to be referred to as: _____

General Practitioner: _____

Community Resources (DN, HV, Social Worker etc.) _____

Previous illnesses: _____

Previous hospitalisation: _____

Work: _____

Recreational Activities: _____

Pets: _____

Allergies: _____

Medications: _____

Prosthesis: _____

Life-style (Parent, family, number of children, religion and home)
Ethnic background:

_____

_____

Typical day profile (have patient describe):

_____

_____

Usual way of coping with stressful events in life:

_____

_____

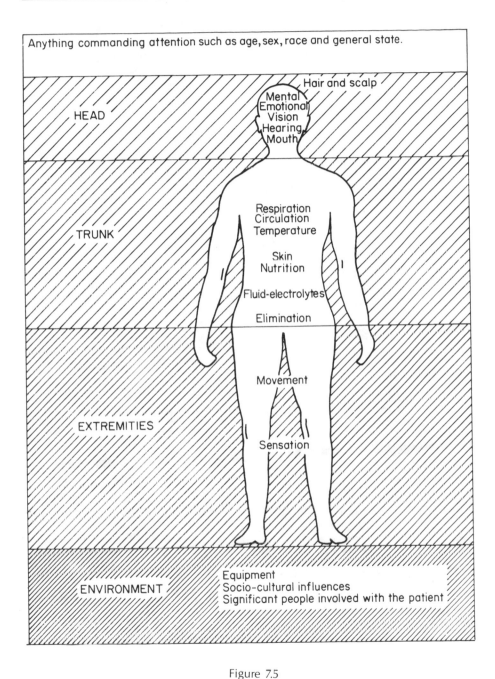

Figure 7.5

It must be stressed that the level or depth to which the nurse should assess a patient using this modified adaptation approach depends on several factors. For example, much depends on the patient's health state and potential problems. Whatever the length of stay, it is the condition of the patient which is important. A handicapped and ill patient will require the nurse to assess nursing problems in greater depth and detail than someone who is fairly fit and only has a minor problem.

The emphasis, during the assessment of a patient using this model, is directed towards the patient's understanding of and participation in nursing care. Positive and negative behaviour is still assessed, along with the patient's ability to adapt to changes in health state.

Finally, in the words of Jim Leeming a consultant physician who had experienced this approach: 'The integration of this new methodology into nursing practice has to be quite slow and gradual, because documentation has to be designed to suit varying needs of different specialities, nurse education has to be modified and attitudes have to change within nursing as well as in other professions. The justification for the change is that it leads to better nursing care. It leads to more reliable and more critical observations by nurses, which helps doctors with their tasks. And it causes a re-evaluation and updating of the contributions of the various professions to patient care'.

References

Beland I L & Passos J Y (1981) *Clinical Nursing*. New York: MacMillan

Fitzpatrick J & Whall A (1983) *Conceptual Models of Nursing*. Maryland: Brady

Fox D (1970) *Fundamentals of Research in Nursing*. New York: Appleton-Century-Crofts

Lewontin R C (1978) Adaptation chapter in special issue on Evolution. *Scientific American*, **239**(3), 156

McFarlane J K & Castledine G (1982) *The Practice of Nursing Using the Nursing Process*. London: C V Mosby Co

Rambo B J (1984) *Adaptation Nursing*. Philadelphia: W B Saunders Co

Randell B, Tedrow M P & Landingham J V (1982) *Adaptation Nursing*. St Louis: C V Mosby Co

Riehl J P & Roy C (1980) *Conceptual Models for Nursing Practice*. New York: Appleton-Century-Crofts

Roy C & Roberts S L (1981) *Theory Construction in Nursing–An Adaptation Model*. Englewood Cliffs, NJ: Prentice Hall

Roy C (1970) Adaptation: a conceptual framework for nursing. *Nursing Outlook*, **18**(3), 42

Roy C (1976) *Introduction to Nursing: An Adaptation Model*. Englewood Cliffs, NJ: Prentice Hall

Roy C (1980) The Roy Adaptation Model. In *Conceptual Models for Nursing Practice*. New York: Appleton-Century-Crofts

Roy C (1984) *Introduction to Nursing. An Adaptation Model*. Englewood Cliffs, NJ: Prentice Hall

Wagner P (1976) The Roy Adaptation Model: testing the adaptation model in practice. *Nursing Outlook*, **24**(11), 662–685

Models for Nursing
Edited by B Kershaw and J Salvage
© 1986 John Wiley & Sons Ltd.

8

A Stress Adaptation Model in Terminal Care

HUGH CHADDERTON

My aim in this chapter is to describe and explain the Roy adaptation model. I will present a specific application of it in the care of a man terminally ill with cancer of the bronchus, to outline how I became interested in the model and what I have done to develop that interest.

My interest in models dates back to the middle to late 1970's, to what is probably best described as an 'untidy realisation' of the need for coherent nursing theory to guide nursing practice. My lead into the literature was by way of contact with the graduates and undergraduates of the University of Manchester's department of nursing. As a result of these contacts, I borrowed and then bought a copy of Riehl & Roy's *Conceptual Models for Nursing Practice* (1980).

Reading Roy's account of her model, I was excited by the considerable potential it offered for both education and practice. Over the next two years I was to undertake two projects to test my ability to teach the rudiments of it, and then practise using it.

I undertook the first of two small intervention studies in 1981 while I was a tutor in South Manchester, as part of the work for the degree of Bachelor of Education. It comprised a short unit of learning to consider the assumptions behind the model, the framework and terminology, and the possibilities for practice in the UK. It involved meeting a small self-selected group of student and pupil nurses twice a week for five weeks.

The second study was undertaken late in 1982 at a hospice in Greater Manchester, as course work for the then Joint Board of Clinical Nursing Studies course 930, 'Care of the dying patient and his family'. I presented to fellow course members, tutors, and the staff of the hospice a case study of a man I was nursing and for whom I was using the Roy adaptation model as a framework for care.

An overview of the model

The history of Roy's model goes back to 1964, when Sister Callista Roy, then a graduate student at the University of California at Los Angeles, was challenged in a seminar with Dean Dorothy Johnson to develop a conceptual model for nursing practice. Accepting the challenge, she developed and refined a model, putting it into operation in a baccalaureate curriculum at Mount St Mary's College in 1968. Classificatory research by Roy and her students (1971), small quasi-experimental studies by Wagner and by Brower & Baker (1976), work by Starr and by Schmitz (1980), action research by Mastal *et al* (1982) and work by many more faculty and colleagues past and present (Roy 1984) have refined and developed the model.

Its basic assumption is that human beings have biological, psychological and social components to their lives, and respond to stimuli from a constantly changing world using both innate and acquired mechanisms. The responses we make determine our bio-psycho-social health and therefore our position on a health-illness continuum. Nursing has the potential both to influence that position and to help an individual adapt to any particular position. Roy's recent writings place greater emphasis on the human being as an open, interactive, interdependent adaptive system.

The 'stimuli' or 'influencing factors' to which Roy refers are essentially synonymous, but the former is an earlier and the latter a later term. The tendency to use 'influencing factors' in more recent writings seems to be aimed at shaking off the behaviouristic and mechanical overtones of 'stimuli'. Stimuli or influencing factors are classified as either focal, contextual, or residual. Focal stimuli are those that immediately confront an individual, such as pathogenic micro-organisms, bereavement or effective health education. Contextual stimuli may be thought of as contributory stimuli and might include environmental temperature and noise levels, genetic make-up or the person's developmental stage, whereas residual stimuli are all the other stimuli that are not validated, including attitudes arising from earlier experiences.

Whether arising outside or inside the individual, stimuli or influencing factors are handled by two sets of processes. Roy (1976) describes these as the regulator and the cognator. The regulator processes are largely autonomous and carried out by the nervous, hormonal and immune systems, such as the control of blood sugar. Cognator processes are the conscious processes of thought and decision, and the unconscious mental mechanisms.

It is important to note that each individual has a limited range of adaptation to any stimulus; we operate within particular zones (Roy 1984). None of us, for example, can cope unaided with life at sub-zero temperatures in the Arctic Circle, with massive haemorrhage, or with the major changes of war.

The outcome of work by the regulator and the cognator processes is behaviour in four modes: the physiologic, self-concept, role function or mastery, and interdependence modes. Behaviour in the physiologic mode includes the familiar biological functions of respiration, circulation, assimilation and elimination. Self-concept behaviour includes the way we view our physical and personal self, in relation to an ideal self or others. Role function behaviours relate to our age, sex, developmental stage and major and minor personal goals (Nuwayhid 1984). Finally, behaviours in the interdependence mode are the relationships we have with those close to us—our significant others (Tedrow 1984)—and are directed towards affectional adequacy: love, security and belonging.

Roy offers the following guidance on what constitutes adaptation, or an adaptive response, in any mode: 'Adaptive responses are those that promote the integrity of the person in terms of ... survival, growth, reproduction and mastery' (Roy 1984). Earlier, she wrote: 'Adaptation decreases the responses necessary to cope with predominant stimulation, and therefore increases sensitivity to complementary stimuli' (Roy 1970). The author's working definitions are essentially internalisations and modifications of those and other ideas. One view is that adaptive responses create conditions which foster survival, growth, reproduction, and mastery of a particular situation, whereas ineffective or maladaptive responses do not. Another view is that an adaptive response enables an individual to deal with a troublesome stimulus, or make best use of a health promoting stimulus, and then move on to other things. A maladaptive response, such as an addiction, fixates the individual and drains his or her adaptive resources.

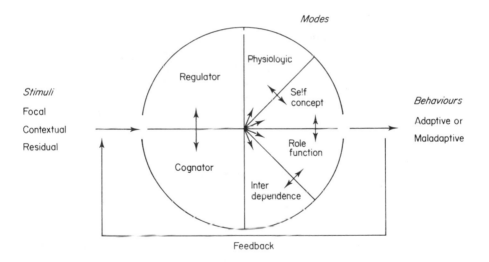

Figure 8.1   The process of adaptation (modified from Roy 1978)

The goal of nursing, stated simply, is to help people adapt to the stimuli that confront them, either by manipulating the stimuli to bring them within their adaptive zones, or by supporting and complementing health-promoting stimuli or responses. Controlling pain and haemorrhage are examples of the former, while praising the efforts of a new father is an example of the latter. The processes of adaptation are illustrated in Figure 8.1.

The five-stage nursing process in the Roy model is described in detail in Roy (1984).

1 The first level assessment

The aim of the first level assessment is the identification of the patient's adaptive and ineffective/maladaptive behaviours. It involves the nurse using her concepts of adaptation while undertaking a systematic review of functioning in all four modes. In the physiologic mode the assessment might include measurement of the familiar parameters of temperature, pulse and blood pressure, estimation of tissue turgor, inspection of pressure areas and generation of a risk assessment score.

Assessment in the self-concept mode involves enquiry about bodily sensations, including pain and body image; and enquiry into the perception of an ideal self, and the rights and wrongs of being ill. In the role function or role mastery mode assessment involves identification of the patient's primary, secondary and tertiary roles, and in the interdependence mode an assessment of how the patient relates to his or her significant others, and an assessment of their support systems (Tedrow 1984).

The first assessment concludes with the nurse making tentative judgements about the degree of adaptation in each mode.

2 The second level assessment

The aim of the second level assessment is to identify the stimuli or factors that influenced or caused the adaptive or maladaptive behaviour. Three points are of particular significance. Firstly, this stage should not only include the identification of physical pathologies, but must take cognizance of the patient's culture, family, stage of growth and development (Sato 1984). Secondly, the assessment must include a search for those factors which promoted the adaptive or effective responses. And thirdly, joint assessment between doctor and nurse may save time and trauma, and is a skill we should develop. This phase concludes with the establishment of the nursing diagnoses.

3 Nursing diagnoses

Nursing diagnoses are essentially simple summary statements about those problems amenable to nursing interventions. They are probably best stated as the relationship between the response and the stimulus. For example, 'refusal of breakfast tray related to fear of gas pains' (Roy 1980), or perhaps 'breakthough pain arising from an inability to manage analgesic medications'.

4 Care planning

Wagner and her students (1976) have tested the model in respect of care planning in in-patient and out-patient settings. In so doing they have developed Roy's assessment and planning tool. This tool, which I used in a modified form in my study, is shown in Figure 8.2; its use is demonstrated in the case study.

5 Evaluating outcomes

Regardless of the setting, or whether the evaluation is ongoing or summative,

| First Level Assessment | | Second Level Assessment | | | Nursing Diagnoses | Interventions | | Evaluation |
Adaptive	Maladaptive	Focal F	Contextual C	Residual R		Goals G	Approach A	
Physiologic Mode Temperature normal. Pulse 82 reg. Skin intact	Extreme weakness	F. Has spent 3/12 in bed	Co-F. Has not been taking adequate diet C. Wife unable to cope.		Extreme weakness or impaired mobility	G. Return of strength	A. (i) Slow mobilization (ii) Small meals (iii) To feed self (iv) Does not require adapted cutlery or crockery.	
Self Concept Mode Not in pain. No altered bodily perceptions	Inability to view self as participant in own care	F. Diagnosis of his cancer in the Bronchus.	C. The couple's inability to discuss this.	R. Healthy up to beginning of June this year.	Situational powerlessness	G. To assess Frank's abilities. G. To address focal stimulus.	A. When appropriate to join Frank and Elsie to discuss Franks abilities viz a viz his illness.	
Role Function Mode								
Interdependence Mode								

Figure 8.2 The nursing process tool (modified from Wagner et al 1976)

the criteria for a satisfactory outcome are the same: that the patient is adapting or has adapted to the stimuli that confront him or her. 'The patient is no longer fixated on the restrictions imposed on him, but is able to take these things in his stride, and free his energies for other things' (Roy 1980)–which seems highly appropriate in the care of a patient who is terminally ill.

A case study of Frank

Before describing Frank and his illness, I would like to clarify the terms 'case study' and 'terminally ill'.

If we accept the definitions offered by Strauss and Glaser (1970), case histories and case studies are quite different. A case history gives prominence to a story which it tells to the fullest, providing a commentary for explanation. A case study on the other hand does not give prominence to the story, only to those parts of it considered necessary for the verification or generation of theory.

Describing Frank as terminally ill at the time depends entirely on your notion of the term. If we accept that it implies that no further chemotherapy, surgery or radiotherapy could be expected to effect a cure, then Frank was terminally ill. But if we set his illness in an adaptation framework, we see that despite his ineffective and maladaptive responses, his resources were far from spent and that he was able to master the situation in which he found himself with appropriate professional help.

Frank was a tall, genial man. A former sales representative for a paper mill, he had lived most of his life in northern England. As a young man he had been active and athletic, playing cricket and rugby union at county level. In his middle years he suffered from rheumatoid arthritis, but as this resolved with time he was able to go walking in the many country parks in his area with his wife Elsie.

Elsie was a soft-complexioned, mild-mannered lady who did not look her 68 years. A former hairdresser, she owned her own business which she wound up when Frank retired. She appeared devoted to her husband and always ready to do as he requested. There were no children by the marriage, no family, and few friends in their immediate neighbourhood.

Frank was admitted to his district general hospital on June 2, 1982, having suffered a myocardial infarction. This was complicated by heart failure and considerable pulmonary oedema. Three weeks later, when his pulmonary oedema had resolved, a 'suspicious area' was noted on his chest X-ray. The next day his physician recommended that he undergo diagnostic bronchoscopy. This took place on July 2 at a nearby cardiothoracic centre, and a biopsy was taken from the lesion found to be partially obstructing his left main bronchus. A further three weeks passed with Frank remaining in hospital, and on July 21 histological tests confirmed the lesion to be an oat cell carcinoma. He was discharged on July 28.

Frank attended the out-patient department of the regional oncology hospital on August 9. A chest X-ray showed his left hemithorax to be opaque, with mediastinal displacement on the right. No metastases were seen. A pleural effusion was diagnosed and aspirated. At this stage he was described as terminally ill, but was admitted for three days of palliative radiotherapy. He attended the department a month later and was described by a radiotherapist as having 'deteriorated'.

During September and October Frank followed a slow downhill course at home, with Elsie's ability to cope with his illness declining. At the request of their general practitioner the couple were visited by the hospice's liaison sister. Her assessment was most revealing; she wrote, 'The main problem is one of weakness. Has been in bed since August, yet can walk quite well, with help, despite arthritis. Poor appetite, taking little nourishment. Likes to be fed. Wife weary and distraught, bed upstairs, Frank won't have it downstairs. No help from family or neighbours'. She recommended admission. This was accepted by all parties and Frank came into the hospice on October 27.

First and second level assessments were made during the first 36 hours following admission. Data were obtained by physical assessment, from the medical and nursing records, from the night nurses' observations, but most important of all from observations of Frank and Elsie's interaction. The first level assessment identified the following adaptive, ineffective and maladaptive responses:

Physiologic mode

Despite mild heart failure, Frank demonstrated adaptive responses in his cardiovascular, integumental and temperature-controlling systems. He did, however, demonstrate ineffective responses in several forms. He was unable to move unaided from bed to chair; he was anorexic—not associated with pain, nausea, or any identifiable abdominal pathology, but he refused all but a little soup and sweet at mealtimes; he was short of breath on exertion, he slept fitfully and awoke frequently; and he experienced difficulty in using his urinal.

Self-concept mode

Frank's self-concept was not explored exhaustively. He was not, however, to my best knowledge, experiencing pain, discomfort, or altered bodily perceptions. A major maladaptive behaviour did become quite obvious within a few hours of admission; he was clearly unable to perceive himself as a participant in his own care. He was not unco operative, but simply seemed not to know what to do to help himself in any given situation. He appeared overwhelmed by his illness; a behaviour consistent with what Roy (1984) describes as 'situational powerlessness'.

Role function or role mastery mode

This behaviour meant that Frank was able to demonstrate few responses in his role function or role mastery mode. In respect of his secondary role (Nuwayhid 1984) he seemed unable to live the life he had left, which included performing the tertiary roles of eating, drinking, eliminating, grooming and so on.

Interdependence mode

The situation appeared rather desperate, but there was hope in the form of adaptive responses to be found in the interdependence mode. Despite all these problems, with little support at home and a rather skewed contributing and receiving relationship (Tedrow 1984), Frank and Elsie showed considerable care and concern for each other.

I would like now to focus on four of the responses outlined in the first level assessment, taking each through to its evaluation stage. The four I have chosen are Frank's extreme weakness; his situational powerlessness; his inability to care for himself; and the couple's affectional adequacy.

First, then, Frank's extreme weakness. The focal stimulus was seen to be that he had spent almost three months in bed, coupled with the contextual or perhaps co-focal stimulus of inadequate food intake. The possibility that he might be suffering from a myopathy was not excluded until he responded to the measures described. The nursing diagnosis was one of impaired mobility, which in retrospect might have been made more specific. The goal of care was a return of strength, and the approach adopted was slow mobilization until he was tired but not exhausted, and the provision of small appetising meals. At the outset the portions were tiny but always tasty, and served at the appropriate temperature. Much time and trouble was taken to organise his environment so that he was able to cope.

Frank progressively regained his strength, vocal timbre, appetite and mobility. By the beginning of November he was able to feed and wash himself, and walk 10-15 yards with a wheeled walking aid before having to stop and regain his composure. He and Elsie were able to spend time away from his bed.

The focal stimulus of Frank's situational powerlessness was seen to be the diagnosis of an incurable disease, set against the contextual stimulus of a wife unable to face her impending loss, and against a residuum of a fairly healthy and active life. The nursing diagnosis was that of inadequate family coping. The goals were to discuss the abilities he still had in reserve, and when appropriate to discuss the focal stimulus itself. When Frank became physically improved, I would join him and Elsie in the afternoon, and if they seemed willing, I would talk with them about the way Frank saw himself and his abilities in relation to his illness. After several such sessions with Frank talking about 'his illness', he used the words 'the cancer' and then 'my cancer'. The way was then clear for discussion. His first questions were about the palliative power of his radiotherapy, which were answered within the hour by his attending physician. Subsequent sessions focused on his input into his care.

Focusing on the focal stimulus seemed to change it and bring it within his adaptive zones, or perhaps it changed his adaptive zones. Whichever it was, he appeared to begin to cope with the stimulus and was able to release his energies for other activities.

I may have given the impression that Frank's problems were largely due to stimuli other than physical illness, but let me now redress the balance. Frank's failure to care for himself was significantly influenced by the co-focal stimuli of his tumour and his age, the contextual stimuli of two major illnesses, and the residual stimuli of ten weeks in hospital (about which little was known). The goal was for him to care for himself as far as he was able, creating a balance between the need for him to master the situation and his limited range of adaptation. To the best of my knowledge he suffered no undue distress or injury as a result of this active, balanced, and carefully monitored approach.

The stimuli that promoted and maintained Frank and Elsie's affectional adequacy were seen to be their relationship up to the beginning of his illness. The relationship apparently involved much caring and sharing of experiences, and goals of care were to promote and support a relationship in the hospice that allowed both to give and to receive. Elsie was encouraged to make the 10-mile drive to visit Frank each afternoon when the heavy traffic had subsided. Her visits were not passive. When well enough Frank would dress, and the couple would walk around the hospice, with Frank using his aid or on each other's arm, and go to the Garden Room for tea. I would often join them there and encourage them to talk about the pleasure they had from their activities and walks in the country parks, and the possibility of taking Frank out to the Peak District national park.

The satisfaction that the couple derived from their shared activities was there for all to see. The balance of giving (contributive behaviours) and receiving (receptive behaviours) appeared to be being restored.

I left the hospice when my course finished on November 14. Returning a week later, I was pleased to see Frank maintaining progress as described; we sat and talked for a short while. Frank was discharged home a little over a week later. Though I am unsure of the circumstances leading to readmission, I learned that Frank, having spent Christmas with Elsie, was readmitted on January 7 and died there on January 20.

My choice of the Roy model

The Roy adaptation model and its nursing process were chosen for the study because the concepts were consistent with my beliefs about the nature of illness and our responses to it, and because the framework offered considerable scope in acting on these beliefs in the care of the dying. Four of the concepts are highly significant.

Firstly, the Roy model offers a dual focus on both the stimuli and the responses. A single pathological diagnosis was long ago seen to be insufficient as a basis for nursing care; a summary of a patient's or a family's response to illness is essential for a balanced view.

Roy's classification of stimuli or influencing factors also squares with my experience of helping patients cope with such problems as sleeping in hospital, longstanding pain, artificial ventilation, and a change in body image.

Thirdly, the notion that we adapt in four adaptive modes is important for nursing practice. It may help us to understand better our patients' response to illness, and provide us with opportunities to help them or their families adapt to their situation.

Finally, the role of the nurse in influencing the patient's position on the health-illness continuum for the better or, if this is not possible, helping them adapt to a particular position, is consistent with modern hospice philosophy—the active treatment of those pathologies amenable to treatment, while providing symptomatic relief for those conditions which are not.

From our use of the Roy adaptation model, Frank and Elsie were helped to understand their problems better. They were helped to understand that there was no single cause of Frank's weakness; that some influencing factors were not amenable to treatment; and that others such as immobility and reluctance to eat were most amenable to nursing interventions. In the same vein they learned that a stimulus such as the diagnosis of malignant disease caused many problems across the modes, but that addressing it at the appropriate time, with staff support, would bring it within their adaptive range.

The couple were treated as an adaptive unit. When appropriate, Elsie would physically support Frank on their trips around the hospice, while the caring and sharing of former times was encouraged as a strategy to help them through their present problems. When discussing progress with them, emphasis was put on their adaptive as well as their formerly ineffective responses. As the goals were made explicit, the criteria for successful outcomes were clear to everyone; the patient, his wife and the nursing staff were well aware of what needed to be done, and able to recognise when any progress had been made.

The principal problem in using the model lay in the use of its terminology. This was not unduly problematic in day-to-day care, as most of the concepts translate into everyday English, but the presentation in unmodified form generated some misunderstanding. I see this as a problem of adaptation, which I hope will be overcome when the model becomes more widely known and acknowledged as useful in helping our patients adapt to whatever troubles them.

In conclusion, I feel that the Roy adaptation model and the Roy model nursing process offer a simple and conceptually compatible framework for use by British nurses who care for dying people and their families.

References

Brower H T F & Baker B J (1976) Using the adaptation model in a practitioner curriculum. *Nursing Outlook*, **24**(11), 686–689

Mastal M F, Hammond H & Roberts M P (1982) Theory into hospital practice: a pilot implementation. *Journal of Nursing Administration*, June, 9–15

Nuwayhid K A (1984) Role function: theory and development. In Roy C (1984) *Introduction to Nursing: An Adaptation Model*. Englewood Cliffs, NJ: Prentice-Hall, 284–305

Riehl J P & Roy C (eds) (1980) *Conceptual Models for Nursing Practice*. Norwalk, CT: Appleton-Century-Crofts

Roy C (1970) Adaptation: a conceptual framework for nursing. *Nursing Outlook*, **18**(3), 42–45

Roy C (1971) Adaptation: a basis for nursing practice. *Nursing Outlook*, **19**(4), 254–257

Roy C (1976) The Roy Model 'Comment'. *Nursing Outlook*, **24**(11), 690–691

Roy C (1978) *Adaptation Model. Supplementary Material for Nurse Theorist General Sessions*. The Second Annual Nurse Educators Conference, New York, December

Roy C (1980) The Roy Adaptation Model. In Riehl J P & Roy C (1980) *Conceptual*

Models for Nursing Practice. Norwalk, CT: Appleton-Century-Crofts

Roy C (1984) *Introduction to Nursing: An Adaptation Model*. Englewood Cliffs, NJ: Prentice-Hall

Sato M K (1984) Major factors influencing adaptation. In Roy C (1984) *Introduction to Nursing: An Adaptation Model*. Englewood Cliffs, NJ: Prentice-Hall

Schmitz M (1980) The Roy Adaptation Model: application in a community setting. In Riehl J P & Roy C (eds) (1980) *Conceptual Models for Nursing Practice*. Norwalk, CT: Appleton-Century-Crofts

Starr S L (1980) Adaptation applied to the dying client. In Riehl J P & Roy C (eds) (1980) *Conceptual Models for Nursing Practice*. Norwalk, CT: Appleton-Century-Crofts

Strauss A L & Glaser B G (1970) *Anguish: A Case History of a Dying Trajectory*. Oxford: Martin Robertson

Tedrow M P (1984) Interdependence: theory and development. In Roy C (1984) *Introduction to Nursing: An Adaptation Model*. Englewood Cliffs, NJ: Prentice-Hall

Wagner P (1976) Testing the adaptation model in practice. *Nursing Outlook*, **24**(1), 682–685

Models for Nursing
Edited by B Kershaw and J Salvage
© 1986 John Wiley & Sons Ltd.

9

A Model for Accident and Emergency Nursing

MIKE WALSH

The self-care view of nursing that is associated with Dorothea Orem originates with her 1959 description of nursing as 'the giving of direct assistance to a person as required, because of a person's specific inabilities in self-care, resulting from a situation of personal health'. Orem developed this concept in the 1960's and published her model of what nursing should be about in her book *Nursing: concepts of practice* (1971), which has since gone into a second edition (1980).

Bromley (1980) describes self-care as 'a requirement of every person, man, woman and child. When self-care is not maintained, illness, disease or death will occur'. Self-care therefore consists of the person's own activities which maintain life, health and wellbeing, carried out on their own initiative and for which they are responsible.

Orem, like the authors of other models of nursing, makes various assumptions fundamental to her theory, starting with the idea of self-care. She describes it as a learned behaviour that is therefore an essential part of human functioning and development. As an infant grows, so too will its self-care ability. This need for self-care is seen as the prime concern of nursing. Self-care action is needed to prevent illness on the one hand, and to recover from illness or at least cope with it on the other. Nursing is legitimately concerned with the ability of the individual to effect that self-care, rather than seeing the person as a passive recipient of care given by a nurse.

Self-care and accident and emergency nursing

Walsh (1985) sums up the general aim of Orem's model as giving assistance so that patients may meet their own self-care requirements as far as possible. This view of nursing harmonises with many areas of patient care, a striking example being in the accident and emergency department. After treatment, most accident and emergency patients return home, where self-care becomes reality. We are no longer dealing with an abstract nursing theory, but rather the reality of whether an elderly lady can get about her home after having her leg plastered, or whether the parents can care for the burns dressing on their child's hand.

Orem's model is not only suitable for care planning with discharge in mind, but also for planning the actual care in the department and, if needed, care on admission. The model recognises that there is a continuum of self-care ability; some patients are incapable of any self-care, while others may be capable of all their care, requiring only advice and teaching from the nurse. Many lie in between those two poles. Moving patients along this continuum in the direction of greater independence and self-care is therefore a second main aim of nursing.

A wide range of patient conditions that may present in A & E are encompassed in the model, from the young girl in a diabetic coma to a workman who has trod on a rusty nail and requires a course of antibiotics. The former is capable of little or no self-care, while the latter's requirements are entirely self-care after the nurse has given teaching about antibiotics and infection. So Orem's model is well suited for A & E nursing in that it deals with the reality of self-care at home and also encompasses a wide range of patient conditions and their attendant nursing requirements.

Concepts used in the model

Humankind

Human beings are seen by Orem as rational, thinking, biological organisms. As such they are affected by their environment and are also capable of predetermined actions which affect themselves, other humans and their environment. How much control, though, do we really have over our own 'health environment'? We will return to this question later in considering a major criticism of the Orem model.

Health

Self-care activity has been understood in terms of maintaining health or moving towards a state of better health. Coleman (1980) describes how this is seen in Orem's scheme as a series of 'therapeutic self-care demands'. What then is therapeutic self-care, given that it accounts for us maintaining our health or trying to improve it?

For the maintenance of health, Orem considers self-care activity in the following areas as essential, and by so doing gives us a ready-made tool for patient assessment:

* Adequate intake of air, water and food.
* Adequate excretion of waste products.
* A balance between activity and rest, both mental and physical.
* Optimisation of social interaction and solitude.
* Avoidance and prevention of hazards to life and wellbeing.
* Feeling and being normal, thereby avoiding stress.

By practising self-care in these six areas, a person maintains a state of health in normal life. Orem refers to them as 'universal self-care demands'.

We need also to consider how the person copes with illness, disease or injury, ie. a deviation from a state of good health. Logically these mechanisms are known as 'health deviation self-care demands', and taken together with the six universal self-care demands above they give us an excellent format for carrying out our nursing assessment. There are three areas to be considered under the heading of health deviancy. These are human structure—anything from a pressure sore to amputation of a limb or breast; physical functioning—examples relevant to nursing might be a stoma or loss of mobility; and behaviour—is the patient depressed, anxious or confused?

We may therefore add together the demands for self-care under these nine headings to make up the total therapeutic self-care demand, the achievement of which constitutes health, our aim. However, realistically we must accept that it is impossible for many of our patients to achieve total health. Rather we aim to give them the best quality of life possible.

A nursing assessment based on the therapeutic self-care demands listed here would seem the most appropriate place to start our nursing care using the Orem model.

Society and nursing

Chapman (1984) points out that Orem considers society as a basically healthy place, and is sharply critical of her self-care model because no allowance is made for the effect of society in causing illness. All is not for the best in the best of all possible worlds! The Black report on inequalities in health (1982) showed how illness and injury were closely linked to social class. Poorer people consistently have worse mortality and morbidity rates for every disease. Moreover, such a simple social factor as gender exerts a major effect, with men under 60 having nearly twice the mortality rates of women.

Orem's model may be criticised on the grounds that many people cannot control their environments and are unable to practise self-care for social reasons. There are far more powerful forces at work in society than the individual, all of which limit the ability for self-care. A multi-million-pound high-pressure advertising campaign is pitted against the individual's self-care ability to abstain from smoking, to quote one obvious example. Consider the unemployed, unskilled labourer in a town like Hartlepool, where male unemployment is over 30%. What can he do to improve his housing conditions or raise his income to afford healthier food? Does he have the knowledge of what healthy food is? This is particularly crucial to the theory of self-care. Without the knowledge, who can practise self-care?

Chapman is right to ask how many psychiatric nurses have watched helplessly as a patient is discharged to the same social conditions which precipitated his illness. In putting Orem's self-care theory into practice, we must therefore consider carefully the social setting the patient has come from and will return to. An interactionist perspective (seeing things from the patient's point of view) will greatly enhance the practice of the self-care model.

Caley et al (1980) describe Orem's view of nursing as 'the giving of direct assistance to a person when he is unable to meet his own self-care needs'. Nursing care should be continually modified as the person moves towards a greater degree of self-care, with less hands-on nursing. Orem also emphasises an holistic view of the individual; we must concentrate not only on the obvious diseased part of the body, but on the whole person, mentally, physically and socially.

The self-care that an individual needs to practise is called the 'self-care demand', but if they cannot meet that demand a self-care deficit is said to exist. This deficit is the initial target of nursing. We should realise that a key target for nursing action to overcome these deficits must be the family and/or significant others in the person's life. Nursing must seek to enhance the care capability of the family and significant others in the pursuit of self-care.

Reference has already been made to a continuum of self-care demands, from the unconscious patient at one end to a person fully able to carry out all their own care at the other. Orem recognises this spectrum in describing her three systems of nursing. A patient who is unable to practise any self-care is said to fall into the wholly compensatory system of nursing, in which the nurse compensates for the self-care deficits wholly as the patient can do little or nothing for themselves. Where the patient is able to carry out some of their self-care but not all, a partly compensatory nursing system is used; finally, if the patient can carry out all their physical requirements for self-care but needs the nurse as a source of advice, information or counselling, an educative-developmental system is used.

The process of nursing

Having briefly outlined some of the basic assumptions behind the Orem model, I will now look at how this theory can be translated into practice.

Assessment

Nursing begins with the assessment of the patient in order to discover their individual nursing problems. These should be defined in terms of a self-care deficit, ie. where the self-care ability of the person and/or others falls short of their self-care demand. This may happen in any of the six areas of universal self-care demand required for the maintenance of health, or in one of the three areas of health deviancy self-care demand associated with illness. The areas of deficit constitute nursing problems for which we must plan nursing interventions. Clearly stated patient goals are required, but more of this later; suffice it to say for now that for practical A & E use we need to make an assessment quickly and easily.

An immediate strength of the Orem model is that it allows us to do just that, lending itself either to a simple checklist style of assessment with space for more detailed information where relevant, or to a simple descriptive style (Walsh 1985; Caley et al 1980). It can further be used in accident and emergency work in conjunction with a standard care plan which will substantially cut down paperwork but leave scope for individualisation (Registered Nurses Association of British Columbia 1977).

Accident and emergency nurses should be familiar with the ABC of resuscitation (airway, breathing, circulation, consciousness), which is where patient assessment begins. The inability of the patient to care for their airway, to breathe to provide sufficient oxygen, or to maintain an adequate circulation or level of consciousness pose immediate threats to life in accident and emergency, and may all be seen as a failure of self-care.

It is therefore logical to commence patient assessment with Orem's health deviancy self-care demands, starting with function and concentrating on the patient's self-care abilities in these four vital areas. This is especially relevant in the patient presenting with a medical emergency such as a stroke or myocardial infarction.

If we move on in line with Orem and assess structure, we are well placed to see the effects of trauma, such as burns, lacerations or fractures, together with previous surgery such as mastectomy or amputation. An outline diagram of the body may be used together with a checklist.

Finally we assess behaviour, which allows us scope to see the effect of the person's injury or illness on their mental state. The problem may be primarily one of mental health; either way, this third dimension of assessment is crucial.

Moving from the health deviancy assessment to the universal self-care demands, we are in a position to build up a picture of how the person manages at home and the background to the immediate problem that has brought them to A & E–crucial to any discharge plans. Our assessment of the 'balance between solitude and socialisation', for example, may reveal an elderly woman living alone with no immediate family, while assessment of the 'balance between activity and rest' may reveal severe limitations due to arthritis. If such a woman had a fall which X-ray reveals has not produced a fracture, doctors often wish to send her home. However, nursing assessment in A & E may reveal that her walking ability is even more limited through pain; taking this with the rest of the background knowledge gained from our assessment, we may conclude that she could not adequately practise self-care at home. A different nursing intervention than simply phoning ambulance transport to take her home is therefore needed.

Planning

Once self-care deficits have been identified, we set goals for the patient, couched in self-care terms for the sake of consistency; so we can make plans for nursing care.

Orem identifies these self-explanatory actions as legitimate nursing acts; acting for, teaching, guiding, supporting and providing a developmental environment. These are incorporated in whichever of the three nursing systems is chosen for the patient–wholly compensatory, partially compensatory or educative-developmental. The goals must be set in terms of observable patient behaviour, for otherwise nursing care cannot be reliably evaluated.

Reference has already been made to standardised care plans in A & E (Walsh 1985; Registered Nurses Association of British Columbia 1977) and their use is recommended as long as sufficient room is allowed for individualisation. The self-care theme should ensure that whatever care is planned for the patient about to be discharged, it is relevant to the reality of self-care at home.

Implementation

(i) Wholly Compensatory System. In A & E nursing the most obvious example of a patient requiring such care is someone who is unconscious; head injury, drugs overdose and diabetic coma being three common causes. There may also be the person with multiple injuries, or a small infant. In such cases the nurse is largely acting for the patient in meeting their self-care deficits, with cardiopulmonary resuscitation being perhaps the ultimate 'acting for' nursing intervention.

(ii) Partly Compensatory System. Here the patient is able to carry out some but not all of their self-care, so the nurse makes good the self-care deficits. A common example from A & E illustrates the point: a woman of 76, living alone, who has fallen and sustained a Colles fracture of the distal radius. Self-care would in theory mean she should relieve her own pain and immobilise her arm in such a way that the bones unite in the correct position. Clearly she is unable to do this, so there are self-care deficits which are the targets of nursing intervention.

Our health deviancy assessment has revealed her to be in pain and frightened, the source of this being a likely fracture of the radius. The goal is that she will relieve her pain and anxiety within 30 minutes; our interventions consist of helping her to take the analgesics prescribed, helping her to immobilise the fracture by temporary splintage, and explaining what is happening in a clear and friendly way. The next goal involves the long-term immobilisation of the fracture once a medical diagnosis has been reached. Again the nurse acts for the patient by applying a plaster cast, meeting the self-care deficit.

We should now look at potential problems, of which the first is swelling within the cast leading to neurovascular compromise. The goal is that the patient will prevent this, the self-care being elevation of the limb. The nursing intervention consists of applying a sling ('acting for') and explaining why she must keep her arm elevated for the next 48 hours ('teaching'), but the patient herself is actually responsible for this care.

Further potential problems include joint stiffness, pain and failure of the plaster cast. The goals are that the patient will retain full use of joints in the hand and arm, will relieve her pain and will care for the cast so that it functions properly. These goals are couched in self-care terms, which is precisely what is required as she will be at home carrying out self-care. Nursing interventions are largely of the teaching variety, concerning finger exercises, when and how many pain-killing tablets to take, and how to care for the cast.

Assessment of universal self-care demands may show that while the woman normally manages to meet them, the added handicap of an arm in plaster will create self-care deficits. Intervention is therefore indicated – extra support from the home help and meals on wheels, or possibly staying with a relative.

In summary, we have a patient who is able to carry out most of her self-care, but who has specific deficits in certain areas which are met by nursing intervention consisting of either acting for, teaching or supporting. The nursing is practical, effective and tuned in to the requirements of self-care at home. Consideration of the many other conditions seen in accident and emergency work will demonstrate the appropriateness of this method of planning care. In most cases a partly compensatory nursing system will be required, whether the person has a cut finger or a myocardial infarction.

(iii) Educative-Developmental System. The nurse here acts as a teacher or counsellor; the patient is self-sufficient in hands-on care. The accident and emergency nurse has many opportunities to practise this, ranging from advice about immunisation against tetanus and simple first aid to discussion about drug overdoses, alcohol abuse or advice on social matters such as battered women's refuges.

Returning to Chapman's criticisms of Orem's lack of awareness of society as a causative factor in ill health, we can develop this system of nursing to compensate for the weakness. Self-care can only be practised if the individual has the knowledge, material resources and the motivation. There is perhaps little that nurses can do about the material resources, but we can impart knowledge and motivation. Nursing has a clear responsibility to move into health education in a big way, not just one-to-one nurse-patient interactions, but collectively in public campaigns on health issues. Health education is a major component of Orem's model.

Evaluation

Without evaluation of the effectiveness of our interventions in assisting the patient to achieve self-care goals, nursing is not complete. Only if goals are set in terms of patient behaviour can we see if they have been achieved. Discharging a patient who cannot look after themselves is a failure of nursing unless adequate arrangements have been made with the community services and all are aware of the self-care deficits. An unhappy return to accident and emergency is likely otherwise.

In conclusion, Orem's model is an excellent base for accident and emergency nursing, where a major function of the nurse is choosing priorities or triage (Walsh 1985). The model offers a good way of carrying out a speedy assessment that will identify immediate life-threatening problems in an emergency. On the other hand it also offers a sound assessment of the patient's ability to manage at home, another major concern of accident and emergency nursing. If we couple this with the harmony between the theory of self-care and the reality for the patient, we have a sound basis for planning nursing care. This basis is even stronger for having built in a health education component with the educative-developmental nursing system. The model acknowledges the wide range of people who attend accident and emergency departments, from those seeking advice to those who are unconscious and have suffered major trauma; the three nursing systems accurately reflect this diversity.

Orem also offers an excellent model on which to base nursing in many other areas such as the community, rehabilitative services like orthopaedic or geriatric nursing, and surgical nursing. The social dimension of health and an appreciation of the situation from the patient's point of view are, however, essential developments the model requires in future.

The thrust of Orem's model is to make people more responsible for their own health care, an approach mirrored by a growing social recognition that we all need to have more responsibility for our own lives. The powerful forces at work in late 20th-century industrial society render us less and less in control of our lives and our own health, precisely when it is recognised that there are insufficient resources made available by the government for the State to fulfil the responsibility. One way out of this dilemma is a greater emphasis on preventing illness in the first place, and increasing the self-care component of nursing in the second. More far-reaching political changes are also needed, but that lies outside the scope of this chapter.

Orem's model of nursing offers us an exciting challenge. It allows us to define an area of knowledge that is specifically nursing knowledge, as opposed to the leftovers of other professions such as medicine. It allows us to move away from the tradition of obedience and discipline to a regard for patients (and nurses) as thinking, responsible human beings fully involved in rational planning of health care.

References

Bromley B (1980) Applying Orem's self-care theory in enterostomal therapy. *American Journal of Nursing*, February, 245–9

Caley J M *et al* (1980) The Orem Self Care Model. In Riehl J P & Roy C (eds) *Conceptual Models for Nursing Practice*. Norwalk, CT: Appleton-Century-Crofts

Chapman P (1984) Specifics and generalities: a critical examination of two models. *Nurse Education Today*, **4**, 141–143

Coleman L (1980) Orem's self-care concept of nursing. In Riehl J P & Roy C (eds) *Conceptual Models of Nursing Practice*. Norwalk, CT: Appleton-Century-Crofts

Doering K & La Mountain P (1984) Flowcharts to facilitate caring for ostomy patients. *Nursing 84*, Sep/Oct/Nov/Dec

Orem D E (1959) *Guide for Developing Curricula for the Education of Practical Nurses*. Washington D C

Orem D E (1971; 1980) *Nursing: Concepts of Practice*. New York: McGraw Hill

Registered Nurses Association of British Colombia (1977) *Standard Care Planning in ER*. Vancouver: RNABC

Townsend P & Davidson N (1982) *Inequalities in Health–The Black Report*. Harmondsworth: Penguin

Walsh M H (1985) *A & E Nursing: A New Approach*. London: Heinemann

Models for Nursing
Edited by B Kershaw and J. Salvage
© 1986 John Wiley & Sons Ltd.

10

Psychiatric Nursing and a Developmental Model

BLAIR COLLISTER

This chapter examines the use of models in psychiatric nursing in two stages. First, the practical application of theoretical models is discussed using models of mental illness as examples, and focusing on the social interaction approach. The second part describes a developmental model of nursing and its application to psychiatric nursing. Attention is drawn throughout to the need for a model to accord with the nurse's view of practice, and for the model to fit reality. But before discussing the use of models in psychiatric nursing, it is worth commenting on the nature of models themselves, and on their usefulness.

It is fair to say that, although most people are not consciously aware of it, we are all philosophers, theorists and model-builders. We all have ideas of how we can make sense of life in general, and of relationships between things and between us and the environment. Each of us has a model for such things as 'education', 'transport' and 'a career', and these models comprise what we believe are its important elements, its characteristics and the relationships between them. The model would also include notions of its purpose and of our behaviour in relation to it. The model we have helps us to identify important events and to forecast what is likely to occur if certain conditions prevail. In theoretical terms the important elements in a model are called concepts, and are often quite abstract. Intuitively we know what we mean by them, and that meaning is generally shared with others who are important to us.

Turning to nursing models, then, they must include concepts which we think are important to be of use to us, and we should share common ideas about the nature of these concepts. Each of us has a model of nursing which guides our approach to practice, teaching or management in our day-to-day job.

The existence of more than one model of mental illness means that most psychiatric nurses know what it is to work with a variety of approaches, and what this means in terms of positive and negative aspects of practice. Siegler & Osmond (1966) give a good description of several conceptualisations of mental illness, and in general the terms medical-biological, behaviourist, psychoanalytical and social-interpersonal are used to encompass the different frameworks identified. Each of these models has a different focus for observation and assessment of the patient, and whichever one is used will influence the nurse's perception of the way in which the patient responds, for example symptomatology or maladaptive behaviour. Each will also influence the chosen goal of action and the nurse's response to the patient. In short, the model will influence our ability to understand and make predictions about the patient.

The experience that any one model may not work with every patient is probably familiar. In some cases, for example, drugs may fail to control a patient's behaviour but he or she may respond positively in a carefully controlled social environment. This shortcoming may also be true of nursing models. They may not be sufficiently refined or address the concepts important to nurses in a given setting, or else the meaning of the concepts may not be sufficiently clear. Because of this inadequacy of individual models, an eclectic approach is suggested in which significant elements from two or more theoretical models are selected and used as a framework for practice.

To give an example from current psychiatric practice of this pluralist approach, dissatisfaction with the medical-biological model and with psychoanalytical theory led to the development of the social-interpersonal framework. It was held that the social context in which the patient or client existed was ignored by the first two formulations. According to Wilson & Kneisl (1983) the social-interpersonal approach includes elements from three theoretical perspectives. These are sociology, interpersonal theory and general systems theory.

From a sociological perspective, mental illness is seen as deviant behaviour. It is noted that deviance is not a property of the behaviour itself, but a quality attributed to it, a consequence of the application of rules by others. Scheff (1967) goes further by suggesting that mental illness is a label given to deviance that cannot be fitted into any other category, that it is a residual category. Psychiatry is concerned with the social audience rather than the individual, since society defines the deviance.

A significant contribution to the interpersonal aspects of the social-interpersonal framework was made by Sullivan (1953). Here the focus is on the individual in the interpersonal situation. The concern of psychiatry is thus the general social climate, usually in the immediate family.

The third significant feature is the inclusion of general systems theory. I do not intend to expand on this theoretical perspective, but it is interesting to note Altschul's suggestion (1977) that systems theory may be an appropriate framework in psychiatric nursing because of the complexity of the situation experienced by many patients. Systems theory can be criticised in this context, however, since it tends to be reductionist rather than holistic in its view of the person. From Menninger's viewpoint (1963), the central feature of systems theory is homeostasis—human balance. Systems theory can serve the understanding of the interplay of relationship between elements at many levels, from the cell (with cellular changes impairing intellect, reasoning and perception) to the community (where social factors such as poverty or unemployment may produce emotional changes in individuals or groups).

Wilson & Kneisl (1983) suggest, however, that the social-interpersonal approach, with its core of action directed to the individual in a social context, has been criticised by psychiatric nurses who see it as being divorced from the real world. It is viewed as impractical, idealistic and ill suited to the realities of psychiatric nursing. This reality is constrained by lack of time, money and other resources, and by the need for symptom control.

It would thus seem appropriate to examine approaches which would have significance for individual nurses in their day-to-day interactions with individual patients. It has been suggested that each nurse has a model of nursing which works for them. It follows that if a model of nursing put forward by a nurse theorist addresses those aspects of practice which are important to psychiatric nurses, it could be useful for practice, education, management and research.

This raises one other aspect of the usefulness of models in nursing practice, concerning the contrast between the application of theories from other disciplines to nursing practice (a model *for* nursing) and the development of a model based in nursing practice (a model *of* nursing). The social-interaction approach in psychiatric nursing reflects the application of theory from other disciplines, framed by medical practice. However, I propose to examine the relevance of a nursing model for psychiatric nursing. The conceptual framework chosen is that of Peplau (1952), whose developmental model was formulated for mental health nursing. The model will be described and explained, and its implications for the psychiatric nurse discussed.

The Peplau developmental model

The focus of Peplau's model is the personal interaction between the nurse and the patient. Nursing is 'a significant therapeutic interpersonal process' between the nurse and the patient which acts as a maturing force and an educative instrument. From these last two points it emerges that nursing is to do with growth and with teaching, and it is in this sense that development takes place. Through the interpersonal process the nurse and client explore the client's reaction to the circumstances of the health problem.

Two concepts basic to Peplau's model are anxiety and communication. Anxiety is held to be an energy source which is related to development, the driving force which promotes biological and psychological growth. When an individual perceives communication in any form as threatening their biological or psychological security, then they experience anxiety. Initially this may promote effective coping through heightened awareness and enhanced performance. However, an increase in anxiety may interfere with the ability to assess reality and to interpret communication appropriately. As a consequence the person may respond either by becoming preoccupied with the physical manifestations of anxiety and with the anxiety reaction itself, or by withdrawing from the real world.

These responses are regarded as health problems; the consequences of illness, especially going into hospital, cause the person to behave in a way which is characteristic of immaturity. It is in this sense—that of regression—that the central idea of development is demonstrated. To become well again the person must grow out of this immature stage.

Communication is seen as a key element in development. It should be noted that communication is used here in its broadest sense – it is not merely giving instructions or information and not concerned only with verbal communication (see, for example, Sundeen *et al*, 1976). Space does not permit further exploration, but the reader is reminded of its magnitude and implications. The importance of communications to every person becomes apparent if we recognise that it influences our perception of reality, our understanding of others, and our understanding of ourselves.

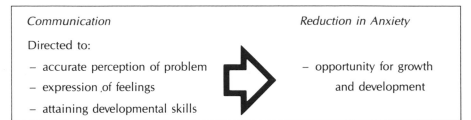

Figure 10.1   The relationship between communication and anxiety (after Peplau 1952)

The relationship between communication and anxiety is depicted in Figure 10.1. Through the intervention of the nurse, the client learns to communicate and be self-aware. The task of the nurse is to promote and maintain a relationship with the patient directed to the goal of reducing anxiety.

The interpersonal process itself receives much attention in Peplau's model. She identifies four phases: orientation, identification, exploitation and resolution.

Orientation

In this phase, the nurse makes the patient aware of the availability of help.

Identification

The nurse facilitates the expression of feelings by the patient, without rejecting them as a person. The patient may respond in one of three ways: as an independent person away from the nurse, as an independent person in relationship with the nurse, or as a person wholly dependent on the nurse.

Exploitation

This is the major working phase of the relationship in which the nurse, through the medium of communication, helps the patient to perceive the problem situation realistically. Growth is then promoted toward the goal of reducing anxiety.

Resolution

In this final phase, the patient disengages from the relationship as an independent person.

Two points arise from this conceptualisation of the interpersonal process. The first is that in a relationship between a particular nurse and patient it may not be possible to progress beyond orientation or identification. The second is that the nature of a particular patient's problem may be such that complete resolution is not possible. The exploitation phase may be continued for some time–perhaps lifelong.

Peplau identifies six roles in which the nurse may engage. Any of these may be adopted throughout the interpersonal process. They are identified in Figure 10.2, and the characteristics shown of the nurse's behaviour in each.

Role	Characteristics
STRANGER	Ordinary courtesy; relate to patient as an emotionally able stranger
RESOURCE	Provide specific answers to questions
TEACHER	A combination of all other roles
LEADER	Establish a democratic relationship with the patient as an active participant
SURROGATE	Assist with resolution of interpersonal conflict
COUNSELLOR	Promote experiences leading to health; increase patient's awareness of needs for health; identify threats to health; facilitate learning through the interpersonal process

Figure 10.2   Roles of the nurse in the interpersonal process (after Peplau 1952)

When engaging in these roles, certain qualities are required of the nurse; firstly that of unconditional acceptance. This reflects a humanistic perspective in which others are valued as individuals and accepted for what they are, and not for what we want them to be. This is an instance of the need for nurses to identify a model which accords with their personal philosophy of life in general and of the worth of others in particular. It leads to the second quality, that of self-awareness. In this context the nurse needs to consider how much of her nursing action is self-directed, and how much she feels controlled by rules, by working in a bureaucratic organisation, or by other health workers.

Thirdly, the nurse needs to maintain an emotional neutrality. She should be able to recognise the response that the patient's behaviour engenders, such as her own anger, anxiety or revulsion. In Peplau's model the nurse is acknowledged as a person, and is expected to understand herself and her reaction to the patient.

This notion of the value of the nurse as a person, and the way in which this idea reflects a particular philosophy of nursing, was one of the prime reasons for selecting this model for discussion.

The central theme of Peplau's developmental model is the interpersonal process, so this is the focus of nurse education. This means not only that the knowledge and skills content of teaching should relate to the interpersonal approach, but also that the principal teaching method should reflect the underlying philosophy. Thus the learner (student or qualified nurse) would be expected to take responsibility for her own development into a practising nurse, with the teacher assuming roles similar to those in Figure 10.2 to facilitate the learner's growth. In addition, the roles of the nurse and the phases of the interpersonal process are each characterised by observable and demonstrable behaviour, which would provide clear objectives for teaching and learning.

These roles and phases also provide a clear definition of the practice of nursing, enabling the nurse to identify the boundaries of nursing and her own skills and learning needs in relation to those boundaries. In selecting a model based on a humanist philosophy, the recognition of the nurse's own philosophy and of the personal qualities inherent in such an approach is of particular importance.

The eclectic approach

These principles are also important if a nurse, group or institution selects elements from more than one model to provide a framework for practice. Some concepts appear intuitively 'right' on first encounter, but subsequently prove difficult as a foundation for practice because of limited applicability, scope or understanding. Experience suggests that activities of daily living (Henderson 1966) and self-care models (Orem 1980) have proved difficult to use in psychiatric nursing as frameworks for assessment or goals of action. Moreover, concepts from different models may not fit together in a pluralist approach because of the perspectives from which they are derived. As an example, it would be inappropriate to attempt to use a developmental or humanistic approach if the nurse or those with whom she worked believed that patients should conform to an institutional routine and had an essentially custodial perspective.

This chapter has sought to examine the use of models in psychiatric nursing, first using familiar examples from psychiatry, and then by describing a model of nursing and its application. Problems encountered when applying a model to practice have been identified. For the most part these could be minimised by appropriate teaching and interpretation on the part of nurse theorists and educators, and even more so by encouraging practising nurses to articulate those concepts—the most important elements—so that a reality-based model could be identified, described and applied.

References

Altschul A (1977) Use of the nursing process in psychiatric care. *Nursing Times*, 73(36), 1412–1413

Henderson V (1966) *The Nature of Nursing.* New York: MacMillan

Menninger K (1963) *The Vital Balance.* New York: Viking

Orem D (1980) *Nursing: Concepts of Practice.* New York: McGraw Hill

Peplau H E (1952) *Interpersonal Relations in Nursing.* New York: Putnam

Scheff T (1967) *Mental Illness and Social Processes.* New York: Harper & Row

Siegler M & Osmond H (1966) Models of madness. *British Journal of Psychiatry,* **112**, 1193–1203

Sullivan H S (1953) In *The Interpersonal Theory of Psychiatry* (eds Perry & Gawel) New York: Norton

Sundeen S, Stuart G, Rankin E & Cohen S (1976) *Nurse–Client Interaction.* St Louis: C V Mosby

Wilson H S & Kneisl C R (1983) *Psychiatric Nursing.* Norwalk CT: Appleton-Century-Crofts

Models for Nursing
Edited by B Kershaw and J Salvage
© 1986 John Wiley & Sons Ltd.

11
A Model for Health Visiting

JUNE CLARK

Disciplines define themselves and distinguish themselves from other disciplines by the particular perspective or frame of reference which they use as the basis for their observations and which in turn directs the form and purpose of their practice. As Luker (1980) points out, 'One of the differences between a health visitor's assessment and that of a hospital or district nurse lies in the theoretical framework upon which she structures her work, and this in turn determines the problems she identifies and hence the goals of her practice'.

Luker's comment presupposes a theoretical framework common to all health visitors and specific to health visiting. Yet health visitors frequently complain that other people do not understand what health visiting is, and other people, notably health service planners, frequently complain that they do not know what health visitors do (Clark 1981). Most experienced health visitors do have an image of health visiting which they use to 'make sense of' what they do as health visitors, and it is this which constitutes their 'model' of health visiting. However, these private images are seldom articulated, and health visiting has yet to formulate any 'theoretical model of health visiting to which all tutors, fieldwork teachers and practitioners subscribe and which they can present to students'—even though the need for this was identified in 1977 by the Council for the Education and Training of Health Visitors (CETHV 1977).

The model presented in this chapter was derived from health visitors' 'private images' as they are presented in the documents of health visiting organisations, and as reflected in the practice of a group of health visitors who taperecorded their home visits and clinic consultations with families for a year as part of a research study (Clark 1985). It has been tested by use in my own practice as a health visitor over two years, but it needs further refinement and testing, especially in work with other client groups.

Why another nursing model?

Why another model, when there are already so many to choose from? And why one specific to health visiting? (In fact this model would be equally suitable for any type of preventive health nursing, and perhaps also for psychiatric nursing.) The answer is that models are a bit like shoes. All shoes are roughly foot-shaped, but if you are on your feet all day you need a pair that fits your particular foot, otherwise you will kick them off under the table as soon as no-one is looking. So it is with models. If the basic concepts and principles are sound, a nursing model can be 'made to work' in any field of nursing. But it may not fit comfortably, and if it does not it is likely, like a pair of uncomfortable shoes, to be discarded. The variation among nursing models arises because each was originally developed in a particular sphere of nursing from the 'private image' of a person whose perspectives, values, and assumptions were inevitably coloured by her own experience. For example Peplau (1952) and Orlando (1961) were clearly influenced by their experience of psychiatric nursing. Differences which on the surface seem slight may reflect quite substantial differences of emphasis in underlying focus and orientation. Such differences are often revealed in practice, in differences in priorities or approaches. There are four places in particular in most nursing models where 'the shoe doesn't quite fit' for health visiting. These are:

1   *The assumption that the focus of care is an individual person*

   The care of a patient must of course take account of the family, but in health visiting the patient usually *is* the family. Health visiting is family nursing, which is described by WHO (1974) as 'based on the concept of the family as a unit and directed to meeting the health needs and concerns of the family'. Clements & Roberts (1983), who asked contemporary nursing theorists to apply their models to family nursing, noted that 'for most of them this is the first time that their theories have been applied to families rather than to individuals. Many of them stated that the exercise was very challenging and in several ways more difficult than they had expected'. Health visiting needs a model in which the focus of care can be a group as well as an individual.

2   *The assumption that nursing is concerned with people's problems*

   This conflicts with the deeply held ideology of health visiting which defines its particular contribution as 'its concern with normal healthy families who do not define themselves as having a problem' (CETHV 1977). Health visitors see themselves as concerned with needs, not problems; they need a model which does not assume the existence of a problem.

3   *The assumption of change*

   The existence of a problem provides a goal for nursing intervention -to remove it, to alleviate it, or in some way to achieve change. Most of the people with whom health visitors work are healthy, and the goal of health visiting is to keep them so–in other words the goal is not change, but stability.

4   *The assumption of a discrete illness episode which begins at the point of admission or referral and ends at the point of discharge*

   Health visiting is a 'serial' activity, that is it takes place over time, often several years, and in such a way that each intervention or interaction is not a new episode but builds upon and is determined by where the last one left off.

A model for health visiting must therefore focus upon the family or group as a unit; needs rather than problems; stability rather than change; and continuity over time. Like any nursing model it must define and relate the key concepts which constitute the paradigm of nursing: person, environment, health and nursing (Fawcett 1983). It must also define and relate concepts which constitute the paradigm of health visiting within nursing: health, prevention, needs and coping (Clark 1985). Health visitors use these terms every day but rarely specify what they mean. The way in which the definitions of these concepts were derived form the health visitors' own use of them is described elsewhere (Clark 1985). The unifying framework which enables them to be linked together in the present model is general systems theory (von Bertalanffy 1968) which has been widely used as a means of understanding the dynamics both of nursing and of families. The person who is the focus of concern (the nurse or the patient, an individual, a family or a community) is seen as a system, that is, a whole which functions as a whole by virtue of the interdependence of its parts; and in particular as an open system, that is a system which affects and is affected by its environment, with which it must maintain a state of balance or equilibrium if it is to survive.
   Within this framework the elements of the model can be defined as follows:

Health is a dynamic equilibrium, a state of balance between the person and his or her environment, in which the balance is held at the level which allows the person to function physiologically, psychologically, and socially at his or her optimum level.
Needs are 'those tangible and intangible items which the person must have in satisfactory amounts in order to attain and maintain ... the physical and psychological balance that we call health' (Johnson & Davis 1975).
Problems. 'If a person's needs are overfulfilled or underfulfilled the balance is disturbed; this disturbance is referred to as a patient problem' (Johnson & Davis 1975).
Coping is the activity by means of which the person strives to maintain equilibrium (the analysis of this concept in this model is based on that of Antonovsky 1979).
Prevention. The model uses the concepts of primary, secondary and tertiary prevention as developed by Caplan (1961) and also used by Neuman (1982). 'By

(primary prevention) I mean the processes involved in reducing the risk that people in the community will fall ill ... The next category of prevention is known as secondary prevention. I use this term to refer to the activities in reducing the duration of established cases of ... disorder and thus reducing their prevalence in the community. Involved here is the prevention of disability by case-finding and early diagnosis and by effective treatment. The last category (tertiary prevention) means the prevention of defect and crippling ... Involved here are rehabilitation services which aim at returning sick people as soon as possible to a maximum degree of effectiveness' (Caplan 1961).

The goal of health visiting–to promote health–is to maintain and over time improve the level of the dynamic equilibrium called health, by heading off harmful stressors and enhancing the client's resistance resources and coping abilities, and by facilitating the entry of beneficial inputs, in the processes of primary, secondary, and tertiary prevention.

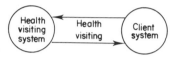

Figure 11.1

The model is shown in diagrammatic form in Figures 11.1 to 11.5. The health visitor and the client are portrayed as two open systems interacting with each other by means of an activity called health visiting (Figure 11.1). This follows Peplau's definition of nursing as 'a significant therapeutic interpersonal process' (Peplau 1952) which was also used by King (1981). Note that the interaction is represented as a two-way process which, following systems theory, affects both systems.

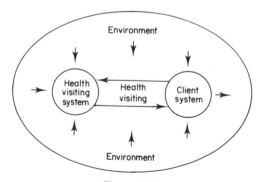

Figure 11.2

The health visiting system may represent the health visiting service or an individual health visitor; the client system may represent an individual, a family, or a community. Each system may contain several subsystems; when the system is a group as opposed to an individual, the only difference in the model is the different set of subsystems which make up the system. The two systems are set within a shared environment with which they constantly interact (Figure 11.2).

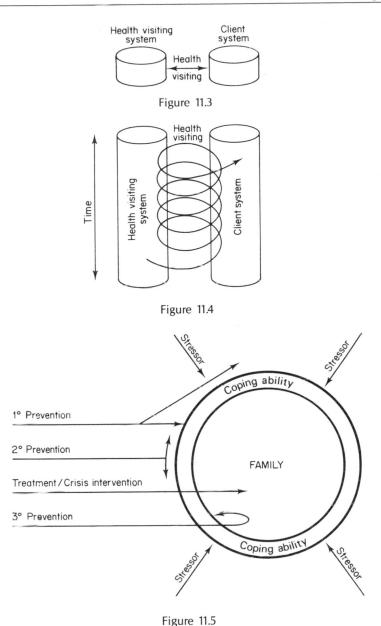

Figure 11.3

Figure 11.4

Figure 11.5

Following Neuman (1982), each of the two systems is represented as a 'core', surrounded by 'rings' which protect the core against harmful stressors while admitting the beneficial inputs which are necessary to meet its needs. When these needs are properly met the system is able to maintain this equilibrium and, over time, to improve the level at which it is held. This is achieved by influencing the stressors which threaten the system's integrity and by building up the client's resistance resources (Antonovsky 1979) and ability to cope with harmful stressors, through the processes of primary, secondary, and tertiary prevention (Figure 11.5).

Figure 11.3 is the same as Figure 11.1 but viewed from a different perspective–that is, it has been turned through 90° from a vertical to a horizontal plane. It is included to show the relationship between Figures 11.1 and 11.4. Figures 11.1, 11.2 and 11.3 show health visiting at a moment in time; figure 11.4 shows a cumulation over time, because as was stressed earlier, health visiting is a 'serial' activity. The significance of Figure 11.4 is that it presents the interaction between health visitor and client not as a series of discrete horizontal lines, but as a continuous spiral in which each twist forms a level higher than the last (ie. later in time) and a continuation of the previous level. Moreover, the three components (the health visitor, the client, and the 'connective' which represents health visiting activity) are not merely in juxtaposition; they interlock with each other like cogwheels or gears, so that each twist of the spiral moves both health visitor and client. This allows the concepts of development and progress over time to be portrayed.

Using the model

The value of a model, however, should be measured not by the way it looks on paper, but by its usefulness in practice. The purpose of the model is to provide a framework for practice. It suggests what kind of information the health visitor should collect in order to make an assessment of the client's needs and to plan and carry out appropriate interventions. This model directs the health visitor to look at the client's needs in terms of the stressors (physiological, psychosocial, environmental, behavioural and developmental) which constitute a potential threat to health equilibrium, and to consider also the resistance resources the client can use to cope with them and thus prevent breakdown. A discrepancy between a stressor and the resistance resources available to cope with it constitutes an actual or potential imbalance in the health equilibrium, ie. a health problem. A simple document which can be used to assess a family's needs and to plan appropriate intervention is shown as used in Figure 11.6 (see below). Modified versions have been developed for use with specific types of client (Clark 1985).

The definition of the problem in turn directs the choice of intervention; for example, an imbalance which is due to lack of knowledge suggests a need for specific teaching as the mode of intervention. The model also encourages identification and analysis of the constraints on various interventions, ie. the stressors which affect the health visiting activity both directly and indirectly through the two systems. Some of the intervention strategies health visitors use are shown in Table 11.1.

A family analysis: the Jones family

The Jones family consists of Ken and Anne Jones and their baby Philip, who was born on February 7, 1984. The first contact between the family and the health visitor was the primary visit on February 17 following notification of his birth. The initial family assessment (Figure 11.6) was recorded at the third visit, on

Table 11.1   Strategies for Health Visiting Intervention

1	*Reducing the client system's contact with harmful stressors by*	
	1.1	reducing or removing the stressor (eg. helping a family to apply for social security benefits)
	1.2	redirecting the client system so that contact is avoided (eg. preventing obesity by teaching about family nutrition)
2	*Improving the client's generalised resistance resources by*	
	2.1	anticipating guidance
	2.2	health teaching
	2.3	developing confidence and self-esteem
	2.4	enhancing general coping behaviour
3	*Improving the client's response to specific stressors by*	
	3.1	anticipating guidance (eg. antenatal classes)
	3.2	specific measures (eg. immunisation)
	3.3	specific health teaching (eg. parentcraft)
	3.4	mobilisation of appropriate resources (eg. referral to a family planning clinic)
	3.5	enhancing specific coping mechanisms (eg. making contact with a support group)
	3.6	support
4	*Systematically surveying the client system for breaches in its integrity by*	
	4.1	specific screening
	4.2	'just checking'
5	*Crisis intervention by*	
	5.1	mobilisation of specific resources (eg. medical referral)
	5.2	supportive counselling
	5.3	practical help
6	*Encouraging reconstitution of the system following breakdown by*	
	6.1	supportive counselling
	6.2	specific teaching

February 28. The assessment/plan forms for Philip were completed when he was two weeks (Figure 11.7) and 14 weeks old; other assessments which were completed later are not included here. Some extracts from the contact record are shown in Figure 11.8.

Using the model to consider the family as a whole as the client system, it can be seen from Figure 11.6 that the major stressors with which it had to cope during this time were Anne's diabetes and the birth of their first child. The family's material and social environment and the couple's own generalised resistance resources were good, and in general they were able to cope successfully with the stressors they had to face. Their equilibrium was maintained and there was no major health breakdown. They remain a normal, healthy family whose generalised resistance resources and level of equilibrium have been enhanced by their success in coping with two major stressors. The family was, however, and still is, potentially at risk of breakdown, and small disturbances of its equilibrium occurred several times.

FAMILY ASSESSMENT/PLAN

NAME . . . . . JONES . . . . ADDRESS . . . 2. SPRINGFIELD ROAD . . . . DATE OF ASSESSMENT 28/2/84

STRESSOR	ASSESSMENT			PLAN	DATE OF CHANGE
	ASSESSMENT OF STRESSOR	RESISTANCE RESOURCES	PROBLEM/NEED		
Physiological	1. Anne: diabetes since 13 yrs., insulin dependent	Good knowledge base, confident self-care	Extra demands of child-birth & lactation	Regular follow-up at diabetic clinic	
	2. Anne: LSCS 7/2/84	No post-op complications	Delay 2nd pregnancy 2 years	Post-natal check at 6/52; contraceptive advice	12/4/84 PN check
	3. Anne: Breastfeeding	Motivation high	Nutrition inadequate	Specialist advice to adjust dietary regime	29/2/84 See contact record
	4. Ken: Susceptibility to asthma	Well controlled, attacks infrequent	Increased risk of allergic response in baby	Watch for infantile eczema	
Psychosocial	1. Young baby, wakeful at night	Stable and mature personalities	Anne is very tired, tense and anxious	Regular supportive visiting	
	2. Both families live 50+ miles away	Bonding is sound			
	3. Inadequate neighbour-hood contacts		Family, neighbourhood contacts inadequate	Introduce to local NCT group	
Environ-mental	Modern semi on new suburban estate. Poor community facilities & public transport	Good material environment Central heating Enclosed back garden	Unguarded gas fire in lounge	Anticipatory guidance 'HIC booklet 'Play it Safe'	
Behavioural	Ken smokes 10+ per day	Anne doesn't smoke and would like Ken to stop	Ken doesn't want to stop	Short term : no smoking in same room as baby. Longer term: Keep under review, fuller assessment needed	9/6/84 See contact record
Develop-mental	First time parenthood No previous experience of small children	Stable marriage 3 yrs. Baby was planned and much wanted. Ken wants to participate in baby's care	Very high expectations of baby and of them-selves as parents	Regular supportive visiting Introduce to local NCT group	
Special needs				Anne has HV's office a'd home 'phone nos. and will contact as necessary	

Figure 11.6 The Jones family: family assessment/plan

CHILD ASSESSMENT/PLAN

NAME .... Philip JONES ..... DATE OF BIRTH .... 7-2-84 ..... AGE .... 14 days ..... DATE OF ASSESSMENT .. 21-2-84 .

BASIC NEEDS	ASSESSMENT		PROBLEM	PLAN	DATE OF CHANGE
	ASSESSMENT	RESOURCES			
Growth	Gest. 37 weeks BW 3160g; HC 34 cm. 50 percentile	Wt. now 3170 g i.e. BW + 10 g		Weigh at home next week. then weekly at clinic	
Normal developmental process - gross motor	Active, moves all limbs, head up when prone; reflexes ✓				
Normal developmental process - hand/eye	Grasp reflex ✓; fixes on mother's face	No risk factors identified	No problems identified	Routine programme of developmental reviews	
Normal developmental process - hearing/speech	Jumps to loud noises				
Normal developmental process - personal/social	Quiets when picked up				
Physical care	Cord off, umbilicus clean & dry, eyes clear	Mother understands care of skin, eyes & umbilicus	Skin around anus is slightly sore	Vaseline as barrier	28/2/84 clear
Nutrition	Breast feeding 3-4 hourly	Baby sucks well; mother's motivation is high		Maintain breast feeding as long as possible NCT contact	
Safe environment	Modern semi on estate - see family form	Central heating at 65°	Large cat; family car is 2 seater sports	To use cat net; to change car, carry cot restraints	10/3/84 new car !
Attachment/emotional security	Bonding with both parents appears sound	Planned and much wanted baby			
Prevention of disease	? full immunisation	Breast fed, no contra indications	Mother unsure about pertussis, wants more info.	Supply leaflets and discuss again next week	10/3/84 consent signed to include pertussis
Special needs				Home visit 28/2/84	

Figure 11.7 The Jones family: child assessment/plan 1

CONTACT RECORD

NAME ....JONES......................... ADDRESS ...2, SPRINGFIELD ROAD

DATE	TYPE OF CONTACT	SUBJECT/ PROBLEM	ASSESSMENT (S/O/A)	ACTION (I)	FOLLOW-UP PLAN (P)	EVALUATION/REVIEW (ER) DATE	
cont. 17/2/84	home visit	Breast feeding	No special instructions given about dietary adjustment	Present diet reviewed Advised increase intake by 400-500 Kc & monitor blood sugar extra carefully	Contact KCH dietician Contact H...P... (diabetic mother who breast fed)	18/2/84	Advised 50g carbohydrate extra, any type, distributed as required
28/2/84	visit	Resumption of intercourse	S ? when to resume - is it necessary to wait 6 weeks ?	Resumption of intercourse, periods, & need for contraception discussed, leaflets given	To contact family planning clinic	9/3/84	Appt. made
14/3/84	clinic	Anne's tiredness	S. feeling very tired, not sleeping well O. tense, near to tears		Home visit late today		
14/3/84	visit	Anne's tiredness	Feeling exhausted in spite of after- noon nap. Baby cries continually, won't settle	Long supportive visit, both parents present. Practical routine discussed. Expectations of parenthood	Anne & Ken will go out for a meal tomorrow, neighbour will babysit	16/3/84	Thoroughly enjoyed themselves- baby cried while they were out then slept all night !
		Feeding while out	Breastfeeding, but baby has had bottle and SMA before	Plan agreed. Breast pump loaned	To feed before leaving & on return.Take breast pump.Leave bottle of water & bottle of SMA in fridge in case	16/3/84	Pump returned - will buy own

Figure 11.8 The Jones family: contact record (extracts)

Health visiting intervention, which was directed by the 'imbalances' revealed by the assessment of stressors and resources, included most of the strategies outlined in Table 11.1. In this case there was no question of avoiding the stressors of Anne's diabetes or Philip's birth; the aim was to enable the family to cope with them in order to prevent breakdown.

Although Anne is normally well able to manage and control her diabetes, and remains 'healthy' even though the disease is constantly present, her health equilibrium was threatened by the physiological demands of pregnancy and childbirth; for example, the reason for her emergency Caesarian section was an acute electrolyte imbalance. The additional demands of breast feeding required adjustment to her diet. The main problem in this case was that Anne's knowledge base was inadequate for her to cope without help. She did not appreciate the need for extra calories during lactation, and did not know how much and what kind of extra food she needed. The health visiting intervention consisted of making Anne aware of her own need, contacting a specialist dietician to find the necessary technical information, sharing the information with Anne, helping her to formulate a new dietary plan, and encouraging her to use it. The maintenance of breast feeding was especially important because of the family history of allergy (Ken's susceptibility to asthma), and this required considerable health visiting intervention in the form of explicit teaching about the physiology of lactation, practical help (experimenting with various feeding positions, lending a breast pump), treatment of an attack of mastitis, and support and encouragement. The intervention was relatively successful in that breast feeding was maintained for 10 weeks, but was finally modified by the additional stressor of Anne's continuing fatigue. At this stage, prevention of a likely breakdown of her own equilibrium was achieved by a new coping strategy – the switch to bottle feeding. This in turn required further health visiting action in the form of teaching and counselling to enable her to come to terms with what she at first saw as her 'failure'. Some of these interventions are recorded in the extracts taken from the contact record, as shown in Figure 11.8.

The couple's ability to cope with the stressors of first-time parenthood required a good deal of support. Their resistance resources as shown in Figure 11.6 were good in that their material resources were more than adequate, their marriage was stable, the baby was planned and very much wanted, and Ken was a supportive and participant father. The problem was Anne's unrealistically high expectations of herself as a mother, and this was exacerbated by her fatigue, which might have been a side-effect of her diabetes or a mild form of postnatal depression. Health visiting intervention was directed to building Anne's confidence in her mothering ability, joint counselling with both parents to modify their perceptions of parenthood and their expectations of their baby, and increasing the availability of social support by introducing them to the local activities of the National Childbirth Trust. Both parents are now much more confident in handling their baby and in identifying and responding to his needs.

After the neonatal period (when all babies of diabetic mothers are especially vulnerable), the baby's health equilibrium has never been in doubt – such is the strength of the human infant's inborn generalised resistance resources. The assessments shown in Figure 11.7 record under several headings 'No problems identified'. In spite of their doubts, his parents have been able to meet all his basic needs. Health visiting intervention has consisted mainly of the strategy of 'just checking', specific screening procedures, and ensuring immunisation against infectious diseases.

Two potential problems which will require further intervention have been identified – Ken's smoking behaviour and Philip's incipient eczema. Philip's skin condition required further assessment which in turn directed an appropriate plan of care (not included here). As Philip grows older, and the couple's ability to cope with parenthood improves, health visiting intervention other than for routine developmental reviews will probably become less frequent. As new stressors and new needs appear (for example the demands of coping with an active toddler as opposed to an immobile baby), and provided that the relationship established so far between client and health visitor is such that Ken and Anne will look to her as one (albeit not the only) source of advice and support, contact will continue. With the passage of time, both client and health visitor will have 'moved on' (as shown in Figure 11.4), and reassessment will be required of the stressors and resources prevailing at the time. Changing circumstances such as a second pregnancy, the collapse of Ken's job or illness in any family member will undoubtedly produce new threats to the family's equilibrium, which will in turn require further assessment, planning and intervention. The goal of health visiting intervention, which will continue for at least the next five years, will be to continue to enhance the family's ability to cope with the stressors with which it will inevitably be presented, and to enable it to achieve normal developmental progress along the family life-cycle.

References

Antonovsky A (1979) *Stress, Health, and Coping*. New York: Jossey Bass

Von Bertalanffy L (1968) *General Systems Theory*. New York: Brazillier

Caplan G (1961) *An Approach to Community Mental Health*. London: Tavistock Publications

Council for the Education and Training of Health Visitors (1977) *An Investigation into the Principles of Health Visiting*. London: CETHV

Clark J (1981) *What do Health Visitors Do? : A Review of the Research 1960–1980* London: Royal College of Nursing

Clark J (1985) *The Process of Health Visiting*. Unpublished PhD thesis. London: Polytechnic of the South Bank

Clements I & Roberts F (1983) *Family Health: A Theoretical Approach to Family Care*. New York: John Wiley

Fawcett J (1984) *Analysis and Evaluation of Conceptual Models of Nursing*. Philadelphia: F A Davis

Johnson M & Davis M (1975) *Problem Solving in Nursing Practice*. Dubuque, Iowa: Wm C Brown & Co

King I (1981) *A Theory for Nursing*. New York: John Wiley

Luker K (1980) *Health Visiting and the Elderly*. Unpublished PhD thesis, University of Edinburgh.

Neuman B (1982) *The Neuman Systems Model: Application to Nursing Education and Practice*. Norwalk CT: Appleton-Century-Crofts
Orlando I (1961) *The Dynamic Nurse Patient Relationship*. New York: Putnam
Peplau H (1952) *Interpersonal Relations in Nursing*. New York: Putnam
World Health Organization (1974) *Community Health Nursing*. Geneva: WHO

12

Looking to the Future

JEAN McFARLANE

We began this book by asking 'Why models?' 'Have they any value in carrying out nursing care?'. We looked at the nature of models and suggested that each of us has an implicit model or paradigm of nursing, its parameters, goals, and methods, which guides our nursing action and that there is benefit in making that model explicit. But in the attempt to do this and to develop conceptual models confusion has arisen. This is not only because there are conflicting models but because the language used to describe them is often imprecise and ill-defined. In addition, many of the models and the literature which describes them have been developed in another culture and whilst there are many commonalities between nursing in North America and the United Kingdom there are many differences. One of the positive features of this book is that nurses practising in the UK have described how they have adapted and developed models and tested them in their own nursing practice. We may now ask, what of the future?

Fashion or permanence?

Are models and their use a nine-day wonder, a fashion, or will they survive in the thinking of the profession with some degree of permanence? I suggest that there is already a permanence about discussions relating to the paradigm of nursing. Miss Nightingale (1859) addressed the question 'Nursing—what it is and what it is not' and indicated that in her view nursing was occupied with the control of the patient's environment so that nature may act upon him or her. But the paradigm has changed from time to time: the Wood report (1947) and the Nuffield Job Analysis of the Work of Nurses in Hospital Wards (1953) gave expression to an implicit model of nursing which was a hierarchy of tasks (basic and technical) relating to body systems and medical treatments. The Platt (1964) and Briggs (1972) reports reflect a different model in which nursing is seen as a team activity directed at holistic and individualised patient care. The focus of nursing care has been stated with increasing clarity as being activities of living, or daily living activities or activities normally undertaken as self care.

At a deeper level of analysis, conceptual models are developed. It is natural that these should undergo change as fashions in theoretical perspectives change. Many of the models reflect dominant concepts and theories developed in other disciplines, eg. interaction, development, systems theory. The models derived from them are useful tools, but they may not reflect the reality or totality of nursing. The models in vogue now need testing and developing, but the use of a model is inherent in the practice of nursing and will continue.

Although the use of models may be inherent and implicit in professional practice, making them explicit and using them intelligently as tools implies a conscious decision to recognise their presence and value and the need for flexibility in practice. Nurses find this far from easy to achieve and it is possible that models may either be adopted and routinised into rigid procedural approaches, or be rejected because flexibility in nursing is too difficult. Models may then become just another fashion because of the inability of nurses to integrate them into a creative and innovative approach to nursing practice. It seems profitable to review some of the very real issues involved in the use of models in practice.

Diversity or dogma?

In this book a diversity of models has been presented. Some would argue that one model is better than another or that one model can lend itself to use in all nursing situations. Educationalists debate the pros and cons of basing the nursing curriculum on one model and the pros and cons of teaching students one model or a diversity of models. Researchers are also concerned to clarify their choice of model. What are the relative positions regarding nursing practice? In the use of a single model one can become competent in using it to guide one's practice, to indicate areas for assessment and the prescription of nursing care. I find, however, in thinking through patients' problems that I frequently employ an interaction model at one point and then move on and think in developmental terms. I may end up using a stress adaptation model or a systems analysis. I use a model and discard it and take up a fresh one very much as an engineer or carpenter uses different tools for different jobs. I suggest that no nursing situation is so simple as to be solely a matter of 'adaptation' or 'development' and nothing else.

Indeed, very few of the models are presented as 'pure models'. Neuman (1985) attributes roots to four main theoretical positions: Gestalt theory, field theories, systems theory and stress adaptation theory. Clark (1985) traces elements of her model to Peplau's (1952) interaction theory, King (1981) and systems theory and Antonovski (1979) as well as Neuman (1985). Orem (1980) draws on role theory, developmental and systems theory. For this reason Thibodeau (1983) describes the Orem model as eclectic (composed of elements drawn from a variety of sources).

This may well represent the reality of nursing. A conceptual model which omits major concepts such as interaction or development may well be an inadequate representation of conceptual relationships in nursing.

Should we be pressing towards a unified model?

Some may feel that there is a need to incorporate some of the established models into a unified model; the time is, I suggest, premature for that. In the first place, some of the models have not been thoroughly tested in practice and there are unresolved philosophical differences between them. Self-care and systems models spring from different philosophical perspectives, their assumptions and values and ideologies are different and they may not readily fuse without prior work to clarify those values and assumptions. Such reservations call into question the legitimacy of eclectic models. Certainly at this stage in theoretical development, it is wise not to allow premature closure of our thinking but to be open-minded about fresh conceptual insights which may be gained from the practice of nursing itself. Unless it be in the self-care/daily living activity models, it could be said that no model yet presented is derived from the practice of nursing *per se* rather than from other disciplines. Stevens (1929) spells out some of the difficulties and questions the search for one right theory and professional conformity; she says, 'It is an attempt to stultify the growth of a discipline'. The attempt to mix or coalesce theory components from numerous authors into a single theory statement assumes that a universal theory is the accumulation of all the pieces of theory done by all known theorists. The problem is that different pieces of theory derive their meaning from their position in a given theory and from their relationship with the components of that theory. Thus, if two nurses use the word 'adaptation' it cannot be assumed to mean the same thing. Therefore, Stevens concludes that attempts at synthesis are futile if taken out of context. Many concepts are incompatible with each other in a logical and meaningful theory statement.

To what extent is there shared meaning?

This leads us to question the extent to which meaning is shared between models using the same words or to what extent different words express the same concepts. To what extent do activities of living, daily living activities and universal self-care needs express the same concepts? Are stressors in the Neuman (1985) model the same as stress in the Roy (1976) model? To what extent have the stages in interpersonal relationships given by Peplau (1952) (articulation, identification, exploitation, resolution) anything in common with the stages of action, reaction, interaction and transaction given by King (1981)? Is the life span concept which Roper, Logan & Tierney (1983) incorporate into their three-way analysis of activities of living, life-span and dependency the same as that used by Rogers (1970)? Not only do the concepts used need to be clarified for their meaning but their relationships and the gaps in the model need to be analysed.

Should there be one model for all fields of nursing?

One may also question whether one model should be used in all fields of nursing. Although it is possible to demonstrate one model being applied in a range of situations, at an intuitive level I find an educational model a better 'fit' for social skill training in mental handicap nursing, and a developmental model a better 'fit' in health visiting and geriatric nursing. But these are personal preferences or preferred tools.

Is it possible to practice, teach or research in a team without an agreed model?

One's personal preferences may be a luxury if one practises nursing as a member of a team – surely some agreement is needed as to the model used? The nursing care of an individual patient needs to be planned and the model of care made explicit so that every nurse involved in the care of that patient will use the same model and care plan. There are, however, different routes to that goal. It may be by adopting a model for use in a particular health authority and providing a conformity of approach and record-keeping and avoiding conflict. Alternatively, different wards may each select a model which is felt to be best suited to their work and use it uniformly for all patients. Lastly, the individual nurse who is allocated a patient may select a model best suited to that patient; in making the care plan she makes the model explicit and all nurses assisting her in the care of that patient use the model. This approach is possible if patient allocation or primary nursing are used as methods of nursing work organisation. The nurse has the autonomy (and is accountable) for the choice of model.

Students working in this situation may find themselves being educated in versatility and creativity, but some educators would plead for the consistent use of one model until the students become competent – which may limit her opportunity to be innovative in her approach to care once she is qualified. Similarly, the researcher working in a team needs to make her model of care explicit so that it can be shared by other members of the team. The solitary researcher also needs to make the model explicit and thereby expose the underlying values and assumptions. The nurse manager has more profound decisions to make about models. Will she facilitate uniformity and easy record keeping and legal accountability, or will she encourage the individual nurse to be creative and make professional decisions about the use of appropriate models for individual patients?

Are we alone in using models?

It is interesting to look, if only briefly, at the use of models by another profession, teaching. Joyce & Weil (1980) review 22 models of teaching which they built into four families of models representing distinct orientations towards people and how they learn (information processing, personal, social interaction and behavioural models). They indicate that a model is a plan or pattern which can be used to shape curricula, to design instructional materials and guide instruction. They point out the 'one right way to teach' fallacy and advocate cultivating a repertoire of models to be used in different teaching situations to accomplish different goals. They indicate how a teacher should develop a repertoire of models (even though it be painful) and give guidance on selection. They suggest that in the first place teachers should become competent in the use of one model from each of the families of models and that this will enrich and add to their teaching style. That seems a parallel situation with our own in nursing! A repertoire of models is desirable for professional practice and students should be encouraged to select one from each of the major families of models.

Conclusions

No one model can ever meet all needs. Every current model requires analysis and evaluation in practice. Most of them are incomplete representations of the reality of nursing and may omit essential features like the goal of nursing action or nursing methods. The concepts themselves, their properties, underlying values and assumptions need explaining. The amount of work to be done and the changes inherent in the adoption of models is not a case for their rejection, however. Without them we lack an essential tool for guiding practice and for making the values and assumptions and goals of our practice explicit–the basis of professional accountability. The profession needs to accept the present lively debate as a challenge to explore our practice and to liberate ourselves from the assumption that there is a right and uniform way to nurse.

References

Antonovski A (1979) *Stress, Health and Coping.* New York: Jossey Bass

Clark J (1985) *The Process of Health Visiting.* Unpublished PhD thesis, Polytechnic of the South Bank

DHSS (1972) *Report of the Committee on Nursing* (Briggs report). Cmnd 5115. London: HMSO

Joyce B & Weil M (1980) *Models of Teaching.* Englewood Cliffs, NJ: Prentice Hall

King I M (1981) *A Theory of Nursing: Systems Concept Process.* New York: John Wiley & Sons

Ministry of Health (1947) *Report of the Working Party on the Recruitment and Training of Nurses* (Wood report). London: HMSO

Neuman B (1985) *The Neuman Systems Model: Application to Nursing Education and Practice.* Norwalk CT: Appleton-Century-Crofts

Nightingale F (1859) *Notes on Nursing, What It Is and What It Is Not.* London: Harrison

Nuffield Provincial Hospitals Trust (1953) *The Work of Nurses in Hospital Wards. Report of a Job Analysis.* London: Nuffield Trust

Orem D (1980) *Nursing: Concepts of Practice.* New York: McGraw Hill

Peplau H (1952) *Interpersonal Relations in Nursing.* New York: Pitman

Rogers M (1970) *An Introduction to the Theoretical Basis of Nursing.* Philadelphia: F A Davis

Roper N, Logan W & Tierney A (1983) *Using a Model of Nursing* Edinburgh: Churchill Livingstone

Royal College of Nursing (1964) *A Reform of Nursing Education* (Platt report). London: RCN

Roy S C (1976) *Introduction to Nursing—An Adaptation Model.* Englewood Cliffs, NJ: Prentice Hall

Stevens B J (1979) *Nursing Theory Analysis Application Evaluation.* Boston, Mass: Little Brown

Thibodeau J A (1983) *Nursing Models: Analysis and Evaluation.* Monterey, Calif: Wadsworth Health Sciences Division

Index